S0-AHA-770

Sexual Maladjustment and Disease:

An Introduction to Modern Venereology

99BB

Sexual Maladjustment and Disease:

An Introduction to Modern Venereology

GAVIN HART, M.D.
Nelson-Hall, Chicago

LIBRARY OF CONGRESS CATALOGING IN PUBLICATION DATA

Hart, Gavin
   Sexual maladjustment and disease.

   Bibliography: p.
   Includes index.
   1. Venereal diseases. 2. Sex deviation.
[DNLM: 1. Sex disorders. 2. Venereal diseases.
3. Sex behavior. WC140 H325s]
RC200.H37   616.9'51   76–29073
ISBN 0–88229–325–7

Copyright © 1977 Gavin Hart

All rights reserved. No part of this book may be reproduced in any form without permission in writing from the publisher, except by a reviewer who wishes to quote brief passages in connection with a review written for broadcast or for inclusion in a magazine or newspaper. For information address Nelson-Hall Inc., Publishers, 325 West Jackson Boulevard, Chicago, Illinois 60606.

Manufactured in the United States of America

Contents

Foreword   ix

Chapter One

Introduction   1
Defining the Problem • Incidence • Neglect and Social
Prejudice • The Future of Venereology

Chapter Two

Sex Education for Health Professionals   11
The Need? • Sexual Health and Sex Education • Sex
Training • *Knowledge* • *Clinical Skills* • *Attitudes* •
Physicians' Roles in Human Sexuality • *Educational
Roles* • *Therapeutic Roles* • *Community Roles*

Chapter Three

Normal and Abnormal Sexual Behavior   19
Normal Sexual Behavior • Sexual Satisfaction and
Venereology • Patterns of Sexual Behavior • *The
Permissive Society* • *Abstinence* • *Premarital Intercourse*
• *Age at First Intercourse* • *Intercourse with Prostitutes*
• *Masturbation* • *Coitus* • *Orogenital Contact* • *Anal
Intercourse* • Sexual Behavior and Venereal Disease •
Abstinence • *Masturbation* • *Coitus* • *Orogenital Contact*
• *Anal Intercourse* • *Significance of Infection Sites*

Chapter Four

Prevention and Management of Unwanted Pregnancy   37
Pregnancy Prophylaxis • *Rhythm Method* • *Condom* •
Hormonal Methods • *Intrauterine Devices (IUD)* •
Sterilization • Management of Unwanted Pregnancy •
Complications of Unwanted Pregnancy • *Techniques for
Termination* • *Complications of Termination* •
Assessment of Unwanted Pregnancy • Bibliography

Chapter Five

Promiscuity and Prostitution   49
     Promiscuity · *Transient Promiscuity* · *Habitual Promiscuity* · Prostitution · *Definition* · *Types of Prostitution* · *Societal Involvement* · *Regulation of Prostitution* · *Repression, Suppression, or Abolition of Prostitution* · *Exploitation of the Prostitute* · *Characteristics of Prostitutes* · *Clients of Prostitutes* · *Function of Prostitution* · *Prostitution and Venereal Disease* · *Conclusions*

Chapter Six

Homosexuality and Homosexual Behavior   73
     Definitions · Homosexuality · *Prevalence* · *Etiology* · *The Psychiatric Status of Homosexuality* · *Management* · Homosexual Behavior

Chapter Seven

The Venereal Diseases   81
     Introduction · *Functional Conditions* · *Urethritis* · *Penile Ulceration* · *Venereal Disease in Women* · *Miscellaneous Conditions* · General Features of the Venereal Diseases · *Age Distribution* · *Sex Distribution* · *Sites of Infection* · *Complication of Pregnancy* · *Coexistence of Several Sexually Transmitted Diseases* · *Evaluation of Sex Partners* · Gonococcal Infection · *History* · *Pathology* · *Clinical Features* · *Diagnosis* · *Treatment* · Nongonococcal Urethritis (NGU) · *Introduction* · *Diagnosis* · *Management* · Herpes Simplex Virus Infection (HSV) · *History* · *Clinicopathologic Aspects* · *Epidemiology* · *Diagnosis* · *Management* · Trichomoniasis · *History* · *Clinicopathologic Aspects* · *Epidemiology* · *Diagnosis* · *Management* · Syphilis · *Introduction* · *Clinical Features* · *Diagnosis* · *Treatment* · Cytomegalovirus Infection (CMV) · Donovanosis (Granuloma Inguinale) · *History* · *Clinicopathologic Features* · *Diagnosis* · *Treatment* · Chancroid (Soft Sore) · *History* · *Clinicopathologic Aspects* · *Diagnosis* · *Treatment* · Lymphogranuloma Venereum (LGV) · *History* · *Clinical Features* · *Diagnosis* · *Treatment* · Pediculosis Pubis · *Introduction* ·

Pathology · *Clinical Features* · *Diagnosis* · *Treatment*
· Scabies · *Introduction* · *Pathology* · *Clinical
Features* · *Diagnosis* · *Treatment* · Corynebacterium
Vaginale Infection · *Introduction* · *Clinical
Features* · *Diagnosis* · *Treatment* · Condyloma
Acuminatum · *History* · *Pathology* · *Clinical Features*
· *Diagnosis* · *Treatment* · Molluscum Contagiosum ·
History · *Pathology* · *Epidemiology* · *Clinical Features*
· *Diagnosis* · *Management* · Candidiasis · *Introduction*
· *Clinical Features* · *Diagnosis* · *Treatment*

Chapter Eight

Environmental and Individual Factors   123
Environmental Stress · Individual Factors · *Race* ·
Age · *Marital Status* · *Education* · *Intelligence* ·
Socioeconomic Status · *Parental Influence* · *Associated
Crime* · *Attitudes and Beliefs* · *Alcohol Intake* ·
Personal Prophylaxis

Chapter Nine

Psychological Aspects of Venereal Disease   141
Personality · Psychosocial Reactions to Venereal
Exposure · *No Reaction* · *Underreaction* · *Overreaction* ·
Clinical Syndromes · *Management*

Chapter Ten

Special Groups   153
Teenagers · Immigrants · The Military · Seamen ·
Individuals Who Do Not Contract Venereal Disease

Chapter Eleven

Failure to Control Venereal Disease   167
Complacency · Treatment Facilities · Influence of the
Medical Profession · Public Attitudes · Female
Reservoir of Infection · Population Mobility ·
High-risk Groups · Immunization

Chapter Twelve

Controlling Venereal Infection   175
Plan or Control Program · *Specialized Coordinating
Staff* · *Clinical Services* · *Epidemiology of Control* ·

*Sensitivity and Specificity · Incidence and Prevalence ·
Disease Control · Attitudes to Disease and Health
Services · Casefinding · Assessing Venereal Disease
Incidence* · Attack Phase · Maintenance Phase
· Eradication Phase · Future Prospects of Venereal
Disease Control

Notes   205

Index   223

Foreword

From personal experience and from discussions with colleagues, I have attempted to provide a unified view of venereology, one apart from the diverse interpretations of the subject in many different environments. It is inevitable, consequently, that the reader will detect many "errors," or views at variance with the accepted "facts" of his own particular scientific environment. This worldwide diversity of opinion is most marked on the relative contribution of physical and psychological factors in venereology. Some will consider I have placed too much and others too little emphasis on psychosomatic aspects.

This book contains many errors of a more absolute nature also. Venereology is awakening from a long hibernation. The disclosures of controlled investigation are rapidly replacing the accumulated dogma of decades. In 1972 an expert venereologist wrote, "Tests of cure are ordinarily not necessary in males, since the cessation of symptoms is usually tantamount to cure [of gonorrhea]."[1] Today this statement would be considered inaccurate, but it was a perfectly reasonable expression of our knowledge a few years ago. Similarly, many of the comments in this book, while presently widely accepted, will fall victim to future wisdom.

However, this is not primarily a book of facts but is rather an approach outlining a human problem. This approach involves a different perspective from that currently held by the majority of health providers. There is little that is new in this book; its uniqueness resides rather in the collection of various components in one volume and in the relative emphasis placed on these components. Furthermore, the author makes no claim for the originality of the outlined concepts, since these have evolved from interaction with teachers and colleagues in different parts of the world over several years. The views expressed are his own, however, and do not necessarily reflect the official policy of any of the institutions with which he has been associated.

Because of differing resources and priorities in different environments, all of the specific services described may not be appropriate in some communities. The general principles, that more attention should be given to the needs of patients, and that health providers should consider broader areas of a patient's sexuality when dealing with specific manifestations of maladjustment, have universal applicability.

Chapter One

Introduction

VENEREAL: "Pertaining to, associated or connected with sexual desire or intercourse"

Shorter Oxford English Dictionary

"Transmitted by sexual intercourse"

Butterworth's Medical Dictionary

Defining the Problem

Venereal disease is a collective term for a group of diverse diseases that have never been rationally delineated and have only one feature in common (sexual transmission). In some countries, the statutory definition includes only syphilis, gonorrhea and chancroid, whereas traditionally Donovanosis (*granuloma inguinale*) and lymphogranuloma venereum (LGV) have been added to this triad. These restrictions are not medically consistent with the literal definition of transmitted during sexual intercourse. Currently there is a tendency to include a wider array of illnesses under the category of sexually transmitted diseases. In the strict sense, a definition of transmission during sexual intercourse is inconclusive, because smallpox and most other infectious diseases also may be transmitted during sexual intercourse. Moreover, the role of sexual intercourse in disseminating candidiasis, trichomoniasis, and gonorrhea, three conditions frequently seen at venereal disease clinics, is distinctly different. From the viewpoint of control, therefore, venereal disease may be defined further as those infections in which sexual transmission is of epidemiologic significance. Table 1-1 lists the major conditions in this category.

1

TABLE 1-1 INFECTIONS FOR WHICH SEXUAL TRANSMISSION IS EPIDEMIOLOGICALLY SIGNIFICANT

Disease	Organism	Size	U.S. Incidence	Complications
Viral				
Herpes genitalis	HSV–2 (DNA virus)	0.2 μ	est. 250,000 annually 200/10^5 adult women	viremia meningoencephalitis eczema herpeticum neoplasia (?)
Condyloma acuminatum	Papova (DNA) virus	0.05 μ	common	
Molluscum contagiosum	Pox (DNA) virus	0.23 x 0.3 μ	unknown	
Cytomegalovirus (CMV) infection	Cytomegalo (herpes) virus	0.2 μ	1–3% newborns 3–5% pregnant women	hepatitis meningoencephalitis ocular infection
Chlamydial				
Chlamydia urethritis, cervicitis	Chlamydia trachomatis	0.25 x 0.5 μ	est. 2 million annually	inclusion conjunctivitis
Lymphogranuloma venereum	LGV (group A Chlamydia)	0.25 x 0.5 μ	report 0.2/10^5	
Mycoplasmas				
?T-mycoplasma urethritis, or cervicitis (unproven)	T-mycoplasma (ureaplasma urealyticum)	0.15 μ	est. 2 million annually	

Disease	Organism	Size	U.S. Incidence	Complications
Larger Bacteria				
Gonococcal infection	Neisseria gonorrhoeae	$0.8 \times 0.6\ \mu$	reported $420/10^5$ pop. est. 2.5 million	PID ca. 15% DGI 1–3%
Chancroid	Haemophilus ducreyi	$0.6 \times 1\ \mu$	reported $0.5/10^5$	
Donovanosis	Donovania granulomatis	$0.6 \times 1.5\ \mu$	reported $0.02/10^5$	
Corynebacterium Vaginitis	Corynebacterium vaginale	$0.5 \times 1.5\ \mu$	est. 15% sexually active population	
Spirochetal				
Syphilis	Treponema pallidum	$0.25 \times 10\ \mu$	reported $24/10^5$ (early and congenital)	Congenital Tertiary
Protozoal				
Trichomoniasis	Trichomonas vaginalis	18–$27\ \mu$	est. 25% sexually active population	
Metazoal				
Scabies	Sarcoptes scabiei	300–$400\ \mu$	common	
Pediculosis pubis	Phthirus pubis	1–4 mm	common	

With the limited resources available, some priority must be established for controlling these diseases. The following factors should be considered, 1) The incidence of the disease (Incidence of those conditions requiring treatment influences both total morbidity from complications and the demand on medical services.), 2) the number and severity of complications, and 3) the cost-benefit of control measures for the various diseases.

Although syphilis has time-honored primacy among venereal diseases, in countries with competent health services it is now virtually confined to underprivileged or socially deprived groups. High prevalence of this infection thus reflects the shortcomings of a particular society rather than the intrinsic nature of disease propagation. Chancroid, Donovanosis, and LGV are known to occur predominantly in tropical or subtropical countries; they have little impact in the United States. Scabies, pediculosis, *Condyloma acuminatum* and molluscum contagiosum may be irritating to the infected individual but are rarely considered serious public health menaces. The total impact of *Corynebacterium vaginale* is uncertain. While cytomegalovirus (CMV) infection has a severe impact on the community, the precise contribution of sexual transmission to this morbidity is unknown. Consequently, current focus among the sexually transmitted diseases should be directed at gonorrhea, nongonococcal urethritis, herpes simplex infection and trichomoniasis (diseases of bacterial, unknown, viral, and protozoal etiologies, respectively).

Expertise in the management of these conditions (*i.e.*, curative skills) forms only part of the tasks of venereologists, since a preventive approach in controlling disease dissemination throughout the community should be the major aim. This control is best directed from control centers—large control facilities with an attached public clinic. Although these clinics must provide excellent medical care, their major role is to provide critical epidemiologic knowledge to disease controllers. This knowledge includes: the contribution to local problems of homosexuality, promiscuity (including prostitution), and recidivism; prophylactic usage; health care acceptance; geographic and sociological high-risk groups. This information can be obtained from all social groups only if the clinic provides convenient and confidential treatment in comfortable facilities operated by a highly competent, sympathetic staff.

For full impact on all social groups, these clinics must meet the needs of the patients and deal either directly or indirectly with their problems relating to sexuality. These problems include

1. Prevention and management of unwanted pregnancy. Sexual health centers should maintain a close liaison with family planning clinics and

when necessary refer patients to these clinics. Where family planning clinics are not readily available, the sexual health center should provide contraceptive assistance. In all settings, however, VD patients should be assessed for the adequacy of their contraceptive protection.

2. Diagnosis and management of all sexually transmitted diseases.

3. Management of psychological and social problems related to infection and some assessment of psycho–social problems related to other aspects of sexuality.

4. Establishment and maintenance of a close personal liaison with all physicians and medical facilities in the area of control.

Developing these control centers and training their staff have priority in control programs for two reasons. The centers may be a prerequisite to controlling venereal disease in some environments. In others, eradication of some venereal diseases may never be feasible. In these circumstances, it is desirable to provide efficient, high-quality ongoing service for patient management.

Directors of these control centers should be specially trained, highly motivated, and keenly interested in human behavior. In addition to a detailed knowledge of the clinical and bacteriologic aspects of the venereal diseases, these physicians must be aware of the attitudes and behavior patterns commonly encountered in the sexually active population. Most important, the physicians must be epidemiologically oriented.

Incidence

"Figures cannot lie, but liars can figure"[1]

Statistics add a stamp of authenticity to any argument, regardless of the inadequacies or deliberate deceptions that may have been involved in their collection and manipulation. Statistics relating to venereal disease are strong contenders for the most inaccurate and misleading original sources of data. A recent national survey in the United States[2] demonstrated that official statistics represented only about 11 percent of the true incidence of venereal disease. Only 10.9 percent of gonorrhea and 12 percent of infectious syphilis cases were reported. This confirmed an earlier survey[3] indicating that only 11 percent of infectious syphilis and gonorrhea were reported. There is no reason to believe that other civilian statistics are any more accurate. They are undoubtedly much less so in many countries with less sophisticated medical services. One source[4] estimates that perhaps only 1 percent of cases may be reported. Military statistics, particularly in wartime, are probably more accurate. The military organization has a tight control over its personnel, and most of the sick are channeled through a unified medical system.

Another source of confusion peculiar to venereal disease statistics is the variable definition of what constitutes venereal infection. In particular, nongonococcal urethritis, which often contributes to as many as 50 percent of cases, has usually been excluded from statistics in the past.

Reported venereal disease has persistently increased in the past two decades. A world health report[4] in 1964 indicated a steady increase in gonorrhea since 1957 in 53 of 111 countries. Total world cases exceeded 60 million annually in 1963. The incidence in the United States is currently estimated at 2 million annually, representing 1 percent of the population.[5] One study on 32,470 women in Chicago showed 5.5 percent to be infected. Of the 9,637 in the 15–19 age group, 6.9 percent were infected.[6] Syphilis is controlled in some countries, although infectious syphilis is considered to be epidemic in the United States. There was a 78 percent increase in reported venereal infection in England and Wales between 1960 and 1969.[7] The incidence in military populations may reach enormous proportions and will commonly grow up to 100 percent *per annum*.[8,9]

Venereal disease currently remains a dominant medical problem in both developed and underdeveloped communities. Furthermore, control of these diseases lags behind that of other medical conditions since it is dependent on social attitudes. With an estimated annual incidence of 150 million, gonorrhea is the most common disease in the world apart from the common cold and childhood infections. Total annual world cases of all venereal infection probably exceed 400 million.

Although these statistics provide a useful impression of the overall magnitude of the problem, more careful analysis of statistics, particularly comparisons of incidence, will usually prove misleading. Paradoxically, when a control program is first instituted and widespread treatment undertaken, the reported incidence of venereal disease may increase quite dramatically despite a mild fall in the true incidence. This occurs because the reduction in infection is of smaller magnitude than the enormous increase in cases disclosed to clinicians. Improved reporting by clinicians may produce a seeming tenfold increase. This one example merely emphasizes the caution required in interpreting changes in reported incidence.

Incidence alone is a poor indicator of total morbidity from a disease. In the Spanish-Portuguese war (1519), over 5,000 penile amputations were performed for VD. It was estimated that the 500,000 cases of syphilis in the French Army in World War I produced 2 million deaths, 157,000 cases of neurosyphilis, and 61,000 cases of cardiovascular syphilis.[10] With modern therapy, these complications are less common, but the psychological sequelae, seen so commonly in modern clinics, may be as distressing as the physical consequences of the past. By reducing such sequelae, the total morbidity of venereal disease may be greatly reduced, although the incidence may remain unaltered.

Neglect and Social Prejudice

> "The medical profession has a long, sad history of lack of interest and of willingness, for the most part, to leave this immense human problem to the less gifted and least high-minded of their brethren."[11]

The causative organisms, method of transmission, adequate diagnostic aids, effective therapy and prophylaxis for both gonorrhea and syphilis are known. Despite this information, which in similar instances has ensured the eradication or control of other infectious diseases, venereal diseases remain uncontrolled. This is because venereal disease is not primarily a medical problem. It is instead a social one dependent on those factors which influence attitudes and behavior, areas where mankind still founders despite considerable sophistication in the biologic and physical sciences. In planning venereal disease control, therefore, we must take into account the frailties and inconsistencies that characterize human nature.

Traditionally, society has regarded sexual behavior other than for reproduction within marriage as degrading. Venereal disease is generally considered to be a sequel of unacceptable behavior and a sign of immorality. Against this background, some may view improvement in the management of venereal disease, whether by providing medical staff, treatment facilities, or by research, as aiding and abetting immorality. This attitude, which still exists in both the lay and medical community, is largely responsible for the current high morbidity from venereal disease. It accounts for the low standing of venereologists, the inadequacy of treatment facilities, and the shame and anxiety still experienced by many patients.

In the past, because venereal disease has been a problem of enormous proportions in military society, more than any other, this institution has dominated the development of venereology. While combat officers have usually advocated aggressive punitive policies, their attitude has also infiltrated military medicine to the point that assignment of medical officers to the treatment of venereal disease has been used as a punitive measure. More importantly, a large proportion of civilian venereologists have been drawn from the military ranks. Many have brought their military attitudes with them. Their clinics more closely resemble a court martial than a place of treatment. An observer could be forgiven for believing that the patient's guilt, rather than his physical and psychological problems, was being assessed.

It should be remembered that during the early training of these older venereologists, venereal disease patients were treated somewhat worse than criminals. During World War I, soldiers with venereal disease in Australia were imprisoned in a barbed-wire enclosure in Victoria (even through World War II, such patients were treated in isolation under armed guard). The "prisoners" were treated as untouchables. They lived in round tents virtually faring for themselves during their confinement, which averaged seven weeks for gonorrhea. The enclosure was guarded by 200 militia, no visitors were allowed, and contact with the outside world was virtually prohibited. In addition to these measures, neither the prisoners nor their families received any pay during the confinement.

After the first six months of this regime, a new camp commandant decided to improve conditions and to restore self respect by building wooden huts and providing adequate drinking water, hot and cold showers, and treatment rooms. To allow some income for them, patients were employed as orderlies. The sequel to this change provides an interesting comparison of punitive versus compassionate therapy (Table 1-2). In the United States, overt punishment of military personnel for contracting venereal disease persisted until 1944.

TABLE 1-2   ABSENTEES (AWOL), DESERTERS, AND MILITARY OFFENCES AT LANGWARRIN HOSPITAL, 1916–1918

Year	Prisoners	AWOL	Deserters	Offences
1916	3161	926	88	1487
1917	1496	199	22	497
1918	793	33	0	108

The reader must not imagine that moralistic condemnation was confined to the military. One doctor wrote to a patient, "You have had the disease one year and I hope it may plague you many more to punish you for your sins and I would not think of treating you."[12] Social prejudice against venereal disease permeates medical thinking, and often it is too subtle to be apparent without some introspection. For example, it is considered appropriate to refer to four patients with syphilis, gonorrhea, Donovanosis, and chancroid as four cases of venereal disease.

To refer to a group of patients with myocardial infarction, emphysema, bronchogenic carcinoma and Buerger's disease as four cases of smokers' disease would be considered a little odd. In both groups the relationship is identical—the four conditions have a common etiologic component. A diagnosis is often written as venereal disease—which, of course, is a moral judgment, not an illness. Paramedical staff commonly refer to a patient with genital pathology (or suspected pathology) as a case of VD when, in fact, only a small proportion of such patients have venereally acquired disease. The degree of moral prejudice and intolerance shown by medical and paramedical staff will be reflected by the impact on the patient. Concealment of disease, illicit treatment, or defaulting are symptomatic of severe intolerance. Lack of cooperation in providing personal information or the names of contacts will occur where rapport is diminished. At an individual level, psychological sequelae following venereal exposure largely reflect inadequate emotional support by the physician. Thus, faulty physician attitudes not only result in large numbers of infected cases being untreated or inadequately treated but aggravate the disability experienced by those persons who are treated.

Because of the social stigma associated with the term *VD clinic*, euphemistic labels have evolved. The name *night clinic* followed naturally from the practice of conducting these clinics in the evening after the respectable outpatients have left the hospital. A storeroom or other makeshift accommodation in the basement was allocated for the purpose, and the unfortunate victim was thrust into the arena by a surly night porter. Surely it is not surprising "now [that] antagonism had developed, cooperation is uncertain and evasion is apparent"[13] when clinics are conducted in this manner.

Special treatment clinic (STC) has had considerable popularity in military environments, although the only special aspect of these clinics was their inferior facilities operated by inferior staff. A waiting room was rarely provided, and the soldiers were forced to queue in the public gaze and endure the derision of their peers.

In fact, the designation VD clinic is inappropriate. Most patients attending do not have venereal disease, and many have no obvious physical illness of any kind. From the patients' viewpoint, however, the deficiencies of past clinics resided not so much in their name but in the conditions created by the way they were conducted. Full patient cooperation is unlikely unless conditions offer complete privacy and maintain the dignity of the individual. Regardless of their name, these clinics should function as sexual health centers and should meet the general sexual health needs of those who patronize them.

The Future of Venereology

"Existing gonorrhea control programs are inadequate, primarily because they do not consider the whole patient."[14]

As the social stigma attached to venereal disease subsides and venereology achieves greater respectability as a medical specialty, marked changes in the role of treatment clinics can be anticipated. Greater emphasis will be placed on treating patients rather than on treating their superficial symptoms. Venereal disease itself may be a relatively insignificant facet of the social and psychological problems confronting a patient. There seems little point in curing his disease without helping him to cope with problems that, if unresolved, are likely to lead to reinfection.

When a patient presents with a number of interrelated problems such as suspected venereal disease, dyspareunia, and contraception difficulties, it is inappropriate to fragment management at several isolated clinics. It is preferable to adopt an integrated approach and consider the overall maladjustment of the individual rather than treating a number of isolated illnesses. The scope of modern venereology, therefore, includes all the psychological, physical, and social problems relating to sexual maladjustment, of which venereal disease is merely one manifestation. This book discusses these aspects of venereology.

Chapter Two

Sex
Education
for
Health
Professionals

The Need?

Traditionally the physician has been assigned the role of chief counselor on matters affecting the physical and mental health of the community. Because of this role and his unique involvement in many intimate problems of his patients, the physician is often assumed to be an expert on sexuality and its manifestations. On the contrary, the physician often has a conservative background. He is further isolated from the realities of contemporary sexual behavior by an extended period of specialized training during which he may have limited contact with society outside his own specialized environment.

The physician may exhibit specific ignorance of sexuality as well as rigid attitudes toward it. Consequently, he is often more ignorant about sexual problems and more uncomfortable in discussing them than the patient. This situation has been perpetuated by the failure of most medical schools to incorporate clinically meaningful training in sexuality into their programs.

This inadequacy is detrimental to the physician's everyday management of his patients.[1] Because of his own embarrassment he often omits a complete sexual history and will avoid breast or genital examinations

11

when these may be critical for adequate management. He rationalizes this avoidance and projects his shortcomings by claiming that such discussion or examination might embarrass the patient. Furthermore, deficiencies in his training leave him ill-equipped to deal with his own sexual feelings which may be aroused periodically by his patients. This may lead to subtle seduction and occasionally to overt sexual behavior. The existence of a hiatus in the physician's training also leaves him inadequate to meet his wider community roles in sexuality, which many consider an important component of his function in modern society.

Sexual Health and Sex Education

A recent World Health Organization paper[2] has defined the concept of sexual health to include:

1. A capacity to enjoy and control sexual and reproductive behavior in accordance with a social and personal ethic.
2. Freedom from fear, shame, guilt, false beliefs, and other psychological factors inhibiting sexual response and impairing sexual relationships.
3. Freedom from organic disorders, diseases, and deficiencies that interfere with sexual and reproductive functions.

This definition has preventive, therapeutic, and training implications. Societal standards and educational goals should be adjusted to remove any barriers to the achievement of sexual health. This applies particularly to the prevention of fear, shame, guilt, and other psychological factors that inhibit sexual response, since these factors stem largely from ignorance, societal taboos, and peer intolerance. Remedial therapy is indicated for individuals who do not meet these criteria of health and who request assistance from their physician. The training given to physicians and other health providers must equip them to provide both appropriate remedial therapy and effective consultation for preventive educational programs.

Many physicians, as well as other members of society, still restrict their view of sexual health to the third component of this definition, and consequently they fail to respond to the needs of their patients who have deficiencies in the other components of sexual health. At a personal level this neglect may result in much needless suffering. Through neurosis, alcoholism, and other deviant behavior, indirectly it may have a devastating effect on society.

Comprehensive training in sexuality is desirable for all counselors in health programs which involve family and marital relations; improvement of maternal and child care; family-life education for school children; treatment of sexually transmitted diseases; and the promotion of mental health. In fact, most of these programs may be considered components of a parent program that deals with psycho-social adjustment. Many of the problems encountered in these fields are manifestations of a more fundamental problem involving sexual maladjustment. The presenting problem cannot be managed adequately without resolving the underlying disorder.

Resistance to the consideration of human sexuality in health programs still persists, nevertheless. For instance, it is sometimes claimed that sexuality training has no role in the control of venereal disease. In fact, some of the deficiencies of the current control program in the United States can be attributed to physicians and other health workers who antagonize patients, particularly homosexuals, because of ignorance, intolerance, or their own sexual anxieties. Homosexuals, who apparently make a large contribution to syphilis morbidity, are reluctant to attend clinics. Those who do attend resist divulging information about their associates who are likely to be infected. Similarly, inability to understand the sexuality of other high-risk groups contributes to diminished rapport with individuals within these groups and impairs their cooperation in disease control.

Sex Training

Adequate sex training involves attention to knowledge, skills and attitudes.

Knowledge

The physician requires a thorough knowledge of biological and psychological sexual development, the reproductive process, and sexual dysfunction and disease. He should also be aware of the variety of sexual expression, the cultural aspects of sex, and how these factors may affect marriage and the family.

In general, past educational programs have adequately covered the biologic and developmental components of this knowledge but have tended to ignore the psychological and sociological patterns. The work of Kinsey, and the research resulting from his initial stimulus, have provided increased insight into both the qualitative and quantitative aspects of sexual expression in Western society. Similar reports from anthropologists make possible cross-cultural comparisons of sexual behavior and its sequelae. Although this knowledge has been poorly disseminated to the medical profession and other health counselors, it is indispensable in providing a perspective for the sexual behavior of an individual or a society. It is inappropriate for an individual to feel shame or guilt about behavior that is practiced by a majority of the population. The prevalence of certain practices in a society or among societies may also influence their acceptance by an individual.

Clinical Skills

The specific clinical skills required by the physician include the ability to recognize sexual difficulty in a reluctant patient. Embarrassment or anxiety frequently prevents a patient from direct presentation with a sexual problem. If the physician is quick to recognize this reluctance, he may minimize the discomfort experienced by the patient. He will often be repaid by increased frankness and cooperation from the patient. Alternatively, the reluctant patient may present with an irrelevant complaint, and without appropriate inquiry from the physician, the real problem will remain undisclosed.

The physician must be able to take a sexual history in a mutually comfortable manner. Most patients are relatively comfortable at providing a sexual history to a competent counselor. Anxiety or uneasiness in the physician, however, are readily transmitted to the patient who often reacts in similar fashion.

The physician should accept the patient as a person and be able to be objective about his sexual behavior. A matter-of-fact approach, showing neither disgust or censure on the one hand nor prurient fascination on the other should be adopted. The physician's own moral standards are irrelevant to the management of the problems of the patient and should not be disclosed, overtly or covertly, as a comparative standard.

The physician must diagnose sexual problems accurately, for this is the keystone to effective treatment. Sexual problems may be complex, and it is sometimes difficult to distinguish secondary manifestations from the primary disturbance. This difficulty is magnified if the patient withholds information or deliberately misleads the physician.

The physician must be prepared to provide effective assistance to the patient. A philosophical discourse may satisfy the physician, but it rarely provides any real benefits to the patient. Definite practical measures must be offered. Therapy must be realistic and tailored to the individual and his social setting. The real test of therapy is to ask two questions. Has therapy decreased anxiety or generally benefited the patient in some way? Has it produced some objective change in behavior which has benefited either the individual or society? If the answer to both these questions is no, worthwhile therapy has not been provided.

An effective referral may be made to provide greater expertise on one facet of diagnosis or management. This greater depth may be achieved at the expense of overall breadth in investigation and management. Once a patient has been channeled into a specialized system, there may be considerable resistance to a change of emphasis in management. For example, psychiatric referral when a physical defect has been overlooked may retard eventual disclosure of the defect because attention has been diverted to psychiatric factors.

Attitudes

Possibly the greatest barrier to the physician's effective management of problems of sexuality stems from his own embarrassment and discomfort. These result from rigid attitudes developed over many years and are consequently difficult to overcome. Many training approaches have been developed for this purpose but none have been subjected to rigorous evaluation. Three techniques have emerged, however, as the most popular for the general physician or health provider. More detailed psychoanalysis or structural analysis may be useful for the specialist, but these are too time-consuming for more general application.

The first of the three techniques privately elicits a student's sex history. The implications of it are then discussed with him. This technique is time-consuming and is very threatening to the participant.

The next technique is group discussion about sexual problems. This is the least threatening of the three techniques and is suited to training large numbers of individuals; however, it enables individuals to evade critical issues of their own sexuality. Unless rigidly directed by an experienced leader, group discussions may degenerate into an exchange of platitudes.

The final technique is the use of explicit sex films. Films showing explicit sexual acts are shown to groups of students who subsequently discuss their emotional reactions to the films. These emotions frequently include sexual arousal, shock, and embarrassment, as well as disgust and hostility.

It is assumed that discussion subsequent to the films desensitizes the participants by dissipating their negative reactions. Such films can also be used to achieve quite specific goals and have unique training potential. They provide a rapid method for detecting specific emotional reactions to certain types of behavior, and they may be the best method of providing insight for the maladjusted counselor. They also have an important role in providing knowledge on sexual techniques.

The degree and type of emotional reaction of any individual to explicit films depend on the type of behavior displayed. This provides a general prediction of the type of counseling situations in which that individual will have difficulty. To provide adequate insight and corrective influence on any participant, it is essential that these emotions are pursued in depth on a personalized basis. Consequently this type of training is best used for small groups of less than 10 individuals. The student should have no trouble in verbalizing his emotions, so there can be no doubt of their existence. This can be followed up by comparing the reactions of the student with those displayed by patients whom the student has previously counseled. The student may complain that the homosexuals he counsels are usually aggressive or hostile, but that he has few problems with other patients. If films of homosexual behavior alone arouse his hostility, it might be argued that the homosexual's hostility merely reflects his own attitudes. This is a simplistic example, of course, but this principle can be used to explore more subtle anxieties or hostilities and demonstrate their role to the student.

A further role of explicit films is to provide comprehensive technical knowledge about practices which are of concern to many patients. Apart from an emotional response that would preclude counseling by most physicians, very few have the technical knowledge to discuss, for instance, methods to maximize the pleasure from and minimize the traumatic or infective sequelae of rectal intercourse or fellatio. Although the use of precoital enemas, anal relaxants, a variety of lubricants, and other techniques are common knowledge to many patients, most physicians are unaware of their existence. Certainly they have no idea of their harm or relative values.

The overall role of sexual training in the medical curriculum is similar to that of the dissecting room. In the one case the student develops a familiarity with the most minute details of human anatomy. At the same time he develops attitudes toward dissection which enable him later to perform surgical procedures with emotional indifference. In the other case, these same attributes are developed for dealing with problems in human sexuality. It might be argued that in both situations the student is exposed to his subject with an indecent degree of intimacy. This probably is necessary if he is to provide a service with an acceptable level of expertise and emotional detachment.

Physicians' Roles in Human Sexuality

The modern physician has educational, therapeutic, and community roles in the field of human sexuality.

Educational Roles

The educational roles of the physician include providing 1) sex education to patients, 2) assistance to parents in understanding their role, 3) assistance to teachers, 4) assistance to young people in understanding their developing sexuality, and 5) premarital assistance regarding sexual adjustment and contraception.

Although the physician must incorporate a degree of sex education into his general management of patients, the major educational efforts in the community must be conducted by parents and teachers. The physician should be qualified to act as an expert consultant for these groups.

Therapeutic Roles

Therapeutic roles of the physician include the management of 1) problems relating to premarital and extramarital sex relationships, 2) unwanted pregnancy, 3) infertility, 4) sexually transmitted diseases, 5) marital disharmony, and 6) so-called deviant sexual behavior.

Since the magnitude of these problems in Western society precludes their routine management by a physician, paramedical personnel may manage the simpler problems and refer more difficult cases to the consultant physician. Specialist clinics also facilitate the handling of large numbers of patients. If these clinics offer care for all kinds of sexual problems, then multiple visits to different facilities are avoided.

Community Roles

The physician should provide advice to community leaders on sex-related problems. Expert counsel is desirable because some "sexual misdemeanors" may respond more readily to therapeutic than to punitive measures.

The mass media should be used responsibly for public sex education. Inappropriate education may produce undue anxiety in the population or inundate clinics with patients who have no need for care. Alternatively, other individuals at high risk for disease, e.g., the asymptomatic contacts of syphilis or gonorrhea patients, may be falsely reassured by the uninformed educator.

The failure of the physician to fulfill these roles has important consequences for both the individual and society. The patient with one sexual problem is at high risk for other sexual problems, and when he visits a health provider he takes all of these problems with him. The promiscuous 19-year old girl who has problems with interpersonal relationships and requests treatment for unwanted pregnancy should be tested for gonorrhea and other sexually transmitted diseases. If she receives a negative reception from the physician, however, she is likely to seek care from nonmedical counselors. Her presenting complaint may be adequately managed, but other important manifestations of her problem will remain undetected. In a similar fashion homosexuals or other categories of persons who are antagonized or cannot receive desired counseling at a clinic will seek treatment from other providers who do not cooperate in disease control programs. For optimum health-seeking behavior by those with sex-related difficulties, it is essential that health providers consider all the related problems which a patient has and then provide meaningful assistance in solving these problems. The primary emphasis must be on the patient's needs rather than on those of the physician. Only when this pattern has been established can we expect meaningful cooperation from patients in alleviating problems of human sexuality (such as venereal disease or unwanted pregnancy) on a community basis.

Chapter Three

Normal
and
Abnormal
Sexual Behavior

Normal Sexual Behavior

"Much depends on whose behavior is being judged, and who is doing the judging."[1]

Defining normality in any branch of science is beset with difficulties, which are compounded in the study of sexual behavior—an involved subject associated with social prejudice and deep-seated moral convictions. Against this background of conflicting opinions and rigid prejudices, we can observe animal behavior and the customs of other human societies to form objective guidelines for normality. To distinguish between normality and abnormality will remain impossible unless we also assess sexual behavior in conjunction with the norms of the society in which this behavior occurs.

Unfortunately, the common criteria for social norms—statutory definition, moral restrictions, societal standards, and actual incidence—are usually conflicting. Normality must be delineated in more general terms. Normal sexual behavior serves an adaptive function and is not associated with undesirable sequelae either to the individual or to society. In modern society, the three adaptive roles of sexual behavior are reproduction, pleasure, and unit solidarity by the strengthening of interpersonal relationships.

Society traditionally has been intolerant of sexual behavior not essential to the reproductive function. Even when associated with this role sexual pleasure has never achieved full respectability. This socially destructive attitude still has many adherents. It is regrettable that in modern times a physician should define sexual deviation as "any mode of sexual behavior which interferes with the functioning of reproduction and in which the sexual behavior has final, persistent preference over normal genital intercourse."[2] At best, this definition implies that human sexual behavior should be relegated to a primitive animalistic role without beneficial psycho-social impact. It also leads to the absurdity of branding as deviant those practices such as contraception which are vigorously advocated by society.

Objective clinical observation indicates that a wide array of sexual behavior is normal since no harmful physical or mental sequelae result. Indeed, those who have a more relaxed attitude and who have indulged in a variety of sexual behavior frequently seem better adjusted and exhibit fewer neurotic manifestations than those who have rigid inhibitions and restrict their behavior to coitus. Associated anxiety and guilt, and compulsive adherence to coitus to the exclusion of other practices indicate abnormal behavior. We should assess sexual behavior as a total entity rather than as a collection of isolated practices. The concept of abnormal sexual behavior is strongly associated with social ignorance and moral convictions, and has little clinical relevance: it is more appropriate to consider the sexual behavior of normal and abnormal individuals. Some practices of very low incidence, such as necrophilia, are probably never performed by normal individuals; possibly they should be considered abnormal behavior. Most behavior, however, cannot be assessed in isolation either from the individuals performing it or the social context in which it occurs. Motivation and psycho-social sequelae to the individual, his partner, and society are more important than physical aspects in delineating normal behavior.

Sexual Satisfaction and Venereology

"Sexual health is mainly involved with flexibility, spontaneity and freedom of preference."[3]

Sexual behavior differs from person to person for several reasons: the sexual drive itself differs; physical and psychological factors modify the sexual drive; and psychological inhibitions influence the expression of the sexual drive. The marked discrepancy in sexual behavior between men and women indicates more than just differences in sexual drive. More men have premarital intercourse; more men engage in nonheterosexual activity; the men who practice these activities engage in them more frequently than corresponding women. These behavioral differences between the sexes are less marked after marriage, however, and vary with social class, being more alike in the higher strata. Such variations suggest that behavioral differences are more a product of attitude and societal standards (particularly the well-established double standard) than sexual drive.

Although the sexual drive is generally considered to vary more between the sexes than it actually does, the sexual drives of two partners may differ markedly. The man frequently has a greater sexual drive, but although it is less publicized, it is probably almost as common for the female partner to have greater sexual drive. Sex differences in sexual drive are further complicated by variations with age. The sexual drive is usually strongest in men in their late adolescence but increases in women into their fourth decade.

The individual need not be concerned about differences between his and his partner's sexual drive. Even large differences are compatible with mutually satisfying sexual adjustment if a genuine relationship exists and if each has a healthy attitude toward sexuality.

Both physical (drugs, fatigue, illness) and psychological factors influence sexual desire. Like all other behaviors, sexual behavior is subject to reinforcement. No doubt women will desire and be willing to indulge practices if these are commonly associated with orgasm. Lack of privacy and the possibility of interruption may decrease sexual performance and pleasure and result in decreasing interest in participation.

However, sexual behavior is remarkable for its flexibility, adaptability, and diversity. For like-minded partners, few physical barriers exist. In a stable relationship with mutual respect, considerable satisfaction may be derived from satisfying the needs of the partner. Although pregnancy, illness, disability, or reduced desire of one participant may preclude any particular activity, there are many alternatives for the sexual fulfillment of one or both partners. By this approach, sexual satisfaction is viewed as a collective product of the union rather than in terms of the desires of the individual participants.

The relevance of this behavior to venereology may be questioned, but its importance lies in its impact on other behavioral patterns. Satisfying sexual relationships are usually exclusive; positive feedback ensures their perpetuation. If diverse behavior is practiced without inhibition, then sexual union develops a highly individualized or specialized character. By satisfying all the sexual needs of the individual, it discourages him from seeking other outlets. In any case, by the very nature of the specialized behavior he has developed over an extended period of time, he loses much of his adaptability for satisfaction in a casual union.

Sexual maladjustment by contrast is conducive to extramarital ventures. If venereal infection then occurs, the physician often becomes involved in an emotion-laden situation. He is subjected to considerable pressure to become an accomplice in deceiving the marital partner. By succumbing to this pressure the physician not only ignores the primary ailment—marital dissatisfaction—but perpetuates the shame and guilt associated with venereal disease. Some unions are so fragile that disclosure may be disastrous. In most situations it is more appropriate to encourage an honest approach that affords both partners the opportunity to ventilate their underlying problems. Instead of providing a solution with a persistent residue of guilt, this policy often produces an overall beneficial outcome by disclosing areas of conflict and by providing methods of coping with these conflicts.

Patterns of Sexual Behavior

The Permissive Society

> "What has changed has been the size of the population engaging in
> certain activities and their greater visibility, not the proportion of young
> people engaging in that behavior."[4]

Today's permissive society is often blamed for increasing venereal disease. Such blame lacks scientific support. Difficult as it is to test experimentally, this hypothesis has not been supported by the studies performed. Promiscuity is the behavioral pattern of primary importance in venereal disease. Despite many claims to the contrary, there is no evidence that this has increased markedly in recent decades. Male behavior has changed little. With continuing emancipation, a greater proportion of women are experiencing premarital coitus but usually with one partner only—the future spouse. This behavior change is therefore irrelevant to the spread of venereal disease.

Although behavior has not changed radically, attitudes have. Nowhere has this change been more obvious than in middle-class Western society. Sex with affection has gained some respectability and is now widely accepted for women as well as men. This increasing frankness and acceptance of sexuality is reflected in more liberal attitudes toward venereal disease, particularly among young people. These attitudes may have increased the reported incidence of venereal disease without increasing the actual incidence, since fewer cases are being concealed or treated illicitly. This increasing frankness and cooperation has had a beneficial effect on all levels of venereal disease control.

The increase in venereal disease and alleged increase in promiscuity have both been attributed to improved methods of contraception—the intrauterine device (I.U.D.) and the pill—but it is doubtful if either of these associations is valid. Coitus between young people, particularly the first experience, is often a spontaneous unpremeditated event that finds both partners unprepared for any form of prophylaxis. By contrast, use of the pill or I.U.D. involves advance preparation. In some ways it indicates a more responsible attitude. Individuals using prophylaxis frequently develop more stable relationships and make no substantial contribution to either promiscuity or venereal disease. The opinion that replacement of the condom with the pill has increased venereal infection unrealistically ignores the fact that condoms have rarely had popularity or significant usage among promiscuous individuals.

Abstinence

"The significance of individual differences is what advocates of abstinence apparently cannot grasp."[5]

Sexual abstinence technically involves refraining from masturbation as well as from sexual involvement with another partner. Furthermore, this absence of sexual outlet occurs concurrently with positive sexual drive and desire for sexual outlet; i.e., there is an element of self-restraint, of combating temptation, or of pleasure denial.

Although it affords protection from venereal disease, abstinence is supported for moralistic, not health reasons. On the other hand, there is the common view among promiscuous groups that abstinence causes physical harm from an accumulation of sexual secretions. The effects of abstinence vary in fact and usually operate through psychological mechanisms. The major factors determining these effects are the sexual drive and temperament of the individual, the duration of abstinence, whether abstinence is enforced or voluntary, and the environment in which it occurs. In young people abstinence may increase sexual desire, with resulting frustrations so distracting that the individual cannot perform his normal work. The psychosomatic sequelae are probably associated with pelvic congestion, manifested as dull pelvic pain or increased glandular secretions of the bowel and genitalia. These symptoms are relieved by masturbation, a practice often unacceptable to the groups that are most prone to these sequelae. Women who have denied themselves intimate contact frequently seem to derive considerable satisfaction from physical examination by the physician.

People hoping to preserve morals or control disease have often unreasonably advocated abstinence for large groups for extended periods. Although it behooves those in authority to counter myths about abstinence and to encourage its application in suitable situations, abstinence is not a feasible alternative to sexual outlet for many individuals in some situations. Consistent with psychological adjustment, masturbation may be preferable to the other sexual alternatives.

Voluntary abstinence is more tolerable if ample opportunities for satisfying physical activity and interesting pastimes are available. It is more difficult to divert the interests of the neurotic, sociopaths, and mentally dull than those of the more adaptable individuals within any group.

Premarital Intercourse

Table 3-1 indicates the variable incidence of premarital intercourse for various groups as studied by several researchers. These studies suggest in general that this behavior is more common in lower socioeconomic sectors, the military, and certain ethnic groups. In environments where coitus occurs between partners of different social classes, the incidence tends toward that for the class of the female partner.

Premarital intercourse by 50 percent of older patients and by 87 percent of younger patients prompted Terman[6] in 1938 to predict that virginity at marriage would be virtually nonexistent for men born after 1930, and that intercourse with a future spouse would be universal by 1950 or 1955. But the proportion of husbands that had premarital sexual relations with a woman other than their spouse has remained stationary (at approximately 50 percent) in the cohorts studied.[7]

Premarital intercourse is now almost universal for men and is experienced by over 50 percent of women. This behavioral change in recent decades is largely attributable to changes in women's attitudes and standards. While the man often initiates sexual behavior, the more conservative, passive woman usually defines the limits of this behavior. Women have increasingly accepted sex with affection, particularly if marriage is anticipated. Most of the dramatic increase in premarital coitus by women has thus occurred with the future spouse. In a recent study of unmarried female undergraduates, 86 percent of those having intercourse did so with a fiancé or steady partner.[8]

Age at First Intercourse

Table 3-2 outlines the age of introduction to intercourse shown by various studies. A study on troops in Vietnam indicated that early intro-

TABLE 3-1 INCIDENCE OF PREMARITAL INTERCOURSE AMONG MEN

Study	%
Kinsey (1948)[a]	
Grade school	94
High school	84
College	68
Hohmann and Schaffner (1947)[b]	
White	79
Grade school	88
High school	81
College	68
Low income	82
High income	75
Jews	84
Catholics	81
Protestants	73
Negro	100
Burgess and Wallin (1953)[c]	68
Landis and Landis (1953)[d]	41
Ehrmann (1959)[e]	
Veterans	73
Nonveterans	57
Seale (1966)[f]	94

[a] Kinsey AC, Pomeroy WB, Martin CE: (1948), Sexual behavior in the human male, 1st ed, WB Saunders, London, 1948
[b] Hohmann LB, Schaffner B: The sex lives of unmarried men, Am J Sociol 52: 501, 1947
[c] Burgess EW, Wallin P: Engagement and marriage, JB Lippincott, Philadelphia, 1953
[d] Landis JT, Landis MG: Building a successful marriage, 2nd ed, Prentice Hall, New Jersey, 1953
[e] Ehrmann W: Premarital dating behavior, Holt and Co., New York, 1959
[f] Seale JR: The sexually transmitted diseases and marriage, Br J Vener Dis, 42: 31, 1966

duction to intercourse was associated with selecting the military as an occupation. Among volunteer soldiers 23 percent had intercourse before 15 years, as compared to 11 percent of the conscript controls ($P < 0.001$).[9] There was a tendency to earlier intercourse with increased family size and less education. Early intercourse also was related to frequency of intercourse in Vietnam (see Table 3-3).

The most striking feature was the marked extroversion ($E = 14.34$) of those having intercourse before 15 and the marked introversion ($E = 10.40$) of those delaying intercourse until after 20. Those first having

TABLE 3-2 CUMULATIVE INCIDENCE OF INTERCOURSE IN VARIOUS STUDIES (Percentages)

Age	1968 Sweden[a] Uni Stud	1968 Sweden[a] Non Stud	1947 USA[b]	1969 Germany[c]	1965 England[d]	1969 Denmark[e]	1971 England[f] VD	1971 England[f] Control	1966 Denmark[g]	1948 USA[h] Grade	1948 USA[h] HS	1948 USA[h] Coll.
9									3			
12					0.5					6	5	1
14	5	20										
15			21	13.1	6							
16	12	50				15.5	30			42	45	9
17			51	47.3	26	49		9				
18	75				34				88	76	74	31
19		100										
20			86	85.3			69	35				
21			93									

a Juhlin L: Factors influencing the spread of gonorrhea. II. Sexual behavior at different ages, Acta Derm Venereol (Stockh) 48: 82, 1968

b Hohmann LB, Schaffner B: The sex lives of unmarried men, Am J Sociol 52: 501, 1947

c Borrmann R: Investigations of preconnubial coition among adolescents in the GDR, in Symp Sexol Prag (Prague) 1969

d Schofield M: The sexual behavior of young people, Longman's, London, 1965

e Hertoft P: Investigation into the sexual behavior of young men, Dan Med Bull [Suppl]. 1: 1, 1969

f Hossain ASMT: Sex behavior of male Pakistanis attending venereal disease clinics in Great Britain, Soc Sci Med 5: 227, 1971

g Ekstrom K: One hundred teenagers in Copenhagen infected with gonorrhea, BR J Vener Dis 42: 162, 1966

h Kinsey AC, Pomeroy WB, Martin CE: Sexual behavior in the human male, 1st ed, WB Saunders, London, 1948

TABLE 3-3 RELATIONSHIP OF SOCIAL FACTORS TO
AGE AT FIRST INTERCOURSE[a]

| | Age at first intercourse | | |
Social Factor	Under 15 %	15-20 %	over 20 %
Over 4 children in family	45.5	35.5	21
Over 3 years high school	29	35	48.5
Intercourse 10 + times in Vietnam	23	23	3

[a] Hart G: The impact of prostitution on Australian troops at war, unpubl doctoral thesis, U Adelaide, South Australia, 1974

intercourse between 15 and 20 were the most stable (N = 9.58) and had an average extroversion score (E = 13.35). Family order and religious beliefs were not related to onset of intercourse. Indulgence in intercourse at an early age suggests future promiscuity and an increased likelihood of contracting venereal disease: 32 percent of those infected compared with 15.5 percent without infection first had intercourse before the age of 15 (P<0.01).[9]

Intercourse with Prostitutes

Patronizing prostitutes is usually confined to a minority of men who have developed normal social relationships, although under extreme stress or during long periods of absence from the normal social environment, most men will seek a prostitute. In a study of soldiers in Vietnam during 1970, all men who attended the VD clinic had also visited a prostitute in the war zone. Of these, 20 percent had visited a prostitute one time in their homeland; 10 percent had done so more than once. In the homeland, patronizing prostitutes was also strongly related to venereal infection: 24 percent of those with a venereal infection in Australia had visited a prostitute more than once; only 8 percent of the uninfected had (P < 0.001). A definite relationship to future promiscuity was also found: of men who had been clients of prostitutes more than once in their homeland, 34 percent had had intercourse more than 10 times in Vietnam; of those who had never been clients, only 17.5 percent had intercourse more than 10 times in Vietnam (P < 0.02).

Kinsey has shown that age and education are related to intercourse with prostitutes (Table 3-4). The most dramatic relationship is the very much lower patronage by those with college education. An almost identical pattern was demonstrated by a random sampling of Australian troops in Vietnam. The proportion of those in Vietnam visiting a prostitute decreased with education: primary education, 75 percent, 1-3 years of high school, 71.5 percent; 4–6 years of high school, 60 percent; and college education, 35.5 percent.[9] This pattern is characteristic of much behavior related to venereal infection; *viz.*, a gradation corresponding to varying degrees of education until the end of high school and then a very great difference for those with higher education. The latter individuals not only have distinctly different behavior patterns but also a much lower incidence of undesirable sequelae from this kind of behavior.

TABLE 3–4 RELATIONSHIP OF AGE AND EDUCATION TO INTERCOURSE WITH A PROSTITUTE[a] (Cumulative Incidence)

Age	Grade	High School	College
20	51	48	21
25	65	63	29
30	70	73	33

[a] Kinsey AC, Pomeroy WB, Martin CE: Sexual behavior in the human male, 1st ed, WB Saunders, London, 1948

Masturbation

> "No other form of sexual activity has been more frequently discussed, more roundly condemned and more universally practiced than masturbation."[10]

Kinsey[11] found the highest incidence (88 percent) of masturbation among single men aged 16 to 20, but 54 percent of the single men at age 50 masturbated (approximately weekly). Among married men, 42 percent of those between 21 and 25, and 11 percent of those between 50 and 60 currently masturbated. Masturbation was related to education; 60–70 percent of college-educated men compared to 29 percent of gradeschool men masturbated after marriage. Furthermore, those with college education masturbated twice as frequently as those with only gradeschool education.

Hohmann and Schaffner[12] found that 90 percent of men with heterosexual experience had masturbated (52 percent currently), whereas 87 percent of virgins had masturbated, and 76 percent still did so at the time of the study.

As Broderick and Bernard[13] indicate, masturbation may be a symptom of many nonsexual conflicts—boredom, frustration, loneliness, poor self-image, conflict with parents, pressure at school, or poor social relations—but it has a useful adaptive function. Among young people it is a component of psychosexual growth. In all groups masturbation provides a release from sexual tension caused by periods of loneliness and sexual deprivation resulting from absence, illness, death, or divorce. The fantasy often associated with masturbation (for 75 percent of males and 50 percent of females) offers a harmless outlet for antisocial urges which, if enacted in real life, would offend the moral code of the individual or society.

Despite the valuable role of masturbation as a sexual outlet that does not involve exposure to venereal disease, it has been violently opposed in the past. Even currently it has limited acceptance.[14] In the past physicians have denounced masturbation, which was claimed to produce a multitude of illnesses, including epilepsy, blindness, impotence, tabes dorsalis, pulmonary consumption, loss of memory, insanity, and even death. Treatment included applying pelvic girdles, binding hands and feet, blistering the penis with mercury ointment, infibulation (insertion of a metal ring through the prepuce), circumcision, sectioning the dorsal nerve of the penis, clitoridectomy, and cauterization of the spine and genitals—surgical mutilation which persisted into the twentieth century.

Most armed forces are hostile to masturbation, evidence of which was once considered sufficient grounds for refusing admission to the U.S. Naval Academy at Annapolis.[15] Nevertheless, universal acceptance of the sentiment that masturbation, "is a normal and healthy act for a person of any age"[16] might well have a favorable influence on the control of VD.

Coitus

By traditional western morals, vaginal intercourse is firmly established as the most desirable marital sexual practice, with extravaginal modes of coitus considered unhealthy, abnormal, or perverse. Of course, to conform completely to this limited definition of normality, a couple must perform even vaginal coitus in only one position and preferably without too much enjoyment. Such an attitude has resulted from the virtually obligatory role of vaginal coitus in reproduction—a traditionally hallowed function that has forced begrudging acceptance (albeit with strictly circumscribed restrictions) of its less reputable precursor.

Vaginal coitus, however, is associated with two very serious hazards —venereal disease and pregnancy. Although venereal disease can also occur with other practices, extragenital infection is less common overall. Pregnancy, while often prized by the married couple, is considered a potential or real disaster in most other social situations. The unhappiness and psychological disturbance resulting from (or from anticipation of) pregnancy or venereal disease have greatly outweighed their physical consequences, though these in themselves have been severe.

In spite of these hazards, coitus has continued to be an important mode of extramarital social expression because of the intense and possibly unique satisfaction afforded by orgasm. Improved methods of contraception have broken the obligatory association of coitus and pregnancy. Both marital and extramarital sexual intercourse for pleasure have gained increasing acceptance. Venereal disease has remained a problem, however.

Indulgence in other sexual practices has demonstrated that vaginal coitus is not the only path to the intense emotional experience related to orgasm. These practices may indeed be more erotically stimulating, provide a more satisfying orgasm, and be practiced in many circumstances where penovaginal intercourse is not possible or practicable. Furthermore, pregnancy is not a potential problem even in the absence of contraceptive action. The chance of venereal infection may be reduced also. There could well be a trend toward further dissociation of sexual behavior and reproduction, so that penovaginal coitus is reserved mainly for definite attempts at reproduction, and other sexual practices are utilized more for satisfaction. Although this would not eliminate venereal disease, total morbidity from the sequelae of sexual maladjustment would be greatly reduced.

Orogenital Contact

In animals, orogenital contact has an important function. Cues of odor, taste, and texture enable the male animal to assess the state of arousal or estrous condition of his mate, and any stimulation to the partner is secondary. In man, orogenital contact is oriented more toward stimulating the partner. The erotic arousal produced in the stimulating partner cannot be denied, and male homosexuals may pay for the privilege of performing fellatio.[17]

Although it is listed as a perversion or abnormality in many textbooks ("Oralism is an attempt to deal with sexuality in terms of breast suckling. . . . it is, therefore, to be regarded as evidence of incomplete development and immaturity"),[18] and is illegal in most of the United States, orogenital acts are used by one-half of all American married couples as part of precopulatory activity (cunnilingus in 54 percent and fellatio in 49 per cent).[19] Ellis considers classification of such acts as a perversion irrational:

It is not any given act of human sexuality that constitutes sex perversion but the psychological motive for which and the consequent inflexible or disorganized manner in which the act is performed.[20]

Sociologically, orogenital acts performed as a part of a continuing relationship should be distinguished from those performed on a casual basis. This was clearly demonstrated by a study on Australian troops in Vietnam.[21] Although 61 percent of troops not sociologically distinguishable from their fellows had experienced fellatio with a Vietnamese prostitute, only 29 percent had done so in their homeland and then almost invariably with a close acquaintance. This practice was much more common among extroverts and the well educated. Kinsey[22] demonstrated a similar relationship between orogenital acts and both education and marital state (Table 3-5).

TABLE 3-5 RELATIONSHIP OF OROGENITAL ACTS TO EDUCATION AND MARITAL STATE

	Before Marriage %	In Marriage %
Cunnilingus		
Grade school	9	4
High school	10	15
College	18	45
Fellatio		
Grade school	22	7
High school	30	15
College	39	43

Among homosexuals, the association between fellatio and the sexually experienced has been demonstrated.[23] In those under 15 years mutual masturbation was the commonest practice (93 percent). Fellatio (50 percent) and anal intercourse (19 percent) were less common. With increasing age, mutual masturbation becomes less common, and fellatio is the major sexual practice (practiced by 84 percent of those aged 15–19).

The desire for fellatio (or oralism in general) is probably a normal component of human eroticism, one that would be indulged more frequently except for the strong inhibitions imposed by conventional Western society. This hypothesis is supported by the widespread practice of fellatio by those individuals for whom conventional taboos prove less restrictive—extroverts, the well educated, and the sexually experienced.

The indulgence of fellatio with prostitutes is a distinctly different phenomenon. Because these contacts are anonymous, societal approval is not a factor. In environments where prostitution forms an important sexual outlet, anonymity is not required since orogenital acts may have high peer acceptance and be viewed more favorably than other sexual outlets such as masturbation. In some areas prostitutes prefer this outlet, which may be technically more convenient and financially more profitable than other sexual acts. Fellatio may be conveniently and quickly practiced in cars,[24] bars, and massage parlors—situations where coitus is more difficult to perform discreetly. This practice is well suited to the mass-output approach by which one girl may, in rapid succession, service a large number of customers in adjacent cubicles.

Orogenital acts owe some of their popularity among both clients and prostitutes to the mistaken belief that they are unlikely to transmit venereal disease. On the contrary, this behavior presents a special epidemiologic problem, for venereal infections in the oropharyngeal region are often asymptomatic. They may remain unsuspected unless specific laboratory investigations are performed. These infections are also more resistant to therapy than those in other areas of the body.

Of 586 patients at one VD clinic, 138 (24 percent) admitted fellatio. Gonococci were cultured from the pharynx of 31 (22 percent) of these. Most of this number were white women whereas most of the clinic patients were black.[25]

Aesthetic considerations have a role in orogenital acts particularly where strangers are involved. The association with education and personality of the man suggests that, although the woman has the less aesthetic role, fellatio is essentially male-initiated. In homosexual relations, however, fellatio is often initiated by the fellator.

Aesthetic factors are even more relevant to cunnilingus. It might be anticipated that this would only be performed on prostitutes or strangers by individuals who could be grouped by certain sociological characteristics. The lower incidence was confirmed by a study in Vietnam that disclosed an incidence of 12.5 percent for cunnilingus compared with 61 percent for fellatio. Although performed by more single than married soldiers (15.5 percent to 4 percent, $P < 0.01$), cunnilingus was not related to a wide variety of sociological parameters of the men. Apparently, therefore, it may be initiated more by the female than by the male partner.

Anal Intercourse

Anal intercourse, while common in homosexual behavior, is not confined to this source. One study indicates that 3 percent of husbands practiced it with their wives.[26] The anus is an erotically sensitive area closely related to the genitalia in both enervation and muscular response. Although anal intercourse may be gratifying to the recipient, considerable experience is probably necessary for the full realization of this erotic potential. A patulous anus that is relaxed on digital examination suggests frequent anal intercourse, but many individuals who periodically indulge this practice have a normal contractile response to examination and a tight sphincter.

Sexual Behavior and Venereal Disease

Abstinence

Because of the specialized adaptation and lability of VD organisms, abstinence affords almost complete protection for the adult. Some individuals refuse, nevertheless, to accept sexual transmission of their disease. They may outline complex mechanisms to implicate the toilet seat, surgical instruments, or other inert intermediaries. The young priest with gonococcal urethritis has acquired his infection venereally regardless of the vehemence with which he may deny this possibility. Medical attendants have only remote risk of infection if they are aware of the high infectivity of all the lesions of early syphilis and pay normal attention to cleanliness. If accidental exposure occurs despite these precautions, treatment should be given as symptoms occur.

Children are not as immune to nonsexual venereal disease as adults, and the parents can infect the child by a variety of routes. *Treponema pallidum* transmitted *via* the placenta may cause abortion, stillbirth, or congenital syphilis in the infant. Both the risk of transmission and the severity of sequelae decrease with the duration of infection in the mother. Gonococcal infection may be acquired during transit of the birth canal. Herpes genitalis poses a serious threat to the fetus. When present at full term, it indicates a need for cesarean section (within six hours of membrane rupture if this occurs).

Gonorrhea, syphilis, and Donovanosis may be transmitted to children by body contact with parents, but sexual transmission should not be dismissed in the very young, whether male or female children and whether the infection is genital or extragenital. Gonorrhea of sexual origin has been reported in three- to nine-year-old children.[27]

Masturbation

Although masturbation is devoid of infective sequelae, the traumatic lesions it commonly produces are susceptible to superinfection on subsequent intercourse. The frenulum is the most common site of trauma, but the prepuce, glans, and corona are also frequently affected. Paraphimosis may occur in the uncircumcised. Trauma and infection may result from foreign bodies inserted into the genital orifices or the rectum, particularly when these become impacted or if glassware breaks. The ingenuity with which individuals explain the presence of the most unlikely objects in the most unlikely places is a source of constant amazement. A foreign body should be considered in the diagnosis of any hard genital mass until direct vision or biopsy indicates otherwise.

Coitus

Contrary to widespread belief among patients, venereal disease is not automatically transmitted during coitus with an infected partner. Gonorrhea is probably transmitted in less than 50 percent of unions between a man and infected woman. Infected men probably transmit gonorrhea in over 50 percent of unions with women. If this were purely a chance phenomenon, a few individuals could be expected to have either very low or very high infection rates after coitus with infected partners. From an epidemiologic aspect, it is important to appreciate that one man may escape infection despite coitus many times with an infected woman when her other concurrent partners may become infected.

It has been suggested that a break in the skin surface is a prerequisite for syphilitic infection, but minor abrasions occur with almost every form of sexual activity. Host resistance is an important factor both in resisting infection and in spontaneous resolution after infection. Infection with *Hemophilus ducreyi* depends even more on predisposing factors. The moist and macerated skin often found beneath the prepuce of the uncircumcised man probably accounts for the much higher incidence in this group than among the circumcised. Lesions occurring in circumcised men or on the shaft of the penis probably result either from a more virulent organism or a diminished host resistance; in practice, these infections are more resistant to therapy. Donovanosis is of low infectivity and is much more common in persons with a poor standard of hygiene.

When transmitted by coitus, herpes genitalis usually results from infection with Herpes simplex virus type 2 (HSV-2). Infectivity is difficult to gauge since genital infection may be quiescent in many individuals. When infection does occur, the incubation period is short (2–20 days, with an average of 6 days). By contrast, genital warts have a longer incubation period (weeks to months) and are of low infectivity.

A high incidence of genital warts is found in the partners of individuals having the disease, but there does not appear to be a significant association between genital and extragenital warts. Trauma may predispose to infection.

Orogenital Contact

Syphilis may be transmitted by oral contact and should be considered in the diagnosis of oral ulcers. Gonorrhea may be transmitted in either direction by fellatio, but the infectivity is unknown. The chance of infection may be considerably less than from penovaginal contact. Infection from pharynx to urethra is probably less likely than in the reverse direction. When a prostitute services a number of clients in rapid succession, the mouth may act merely as an incubator for transfer without pharyngeal infection.

Herpes simplex virus is commonly transmitted by fellatio, which may result in HSV-2 infection of the mouth and occasionally HSV-1 genital infection. These viruses occur at the reverse sites in the preponderance of infections. Severe trauma, particularly in the uncircumcised man, may follow fellatio.

Anal Intercourse

Syphilis and gonorrhea are both readily transmitted by anal intercourse. Repeated anal intercourse may also produce various rectal symptoms, including mucous or mucopurulent discharge, without venereal infection. Rectal symptoms of infected persons are not appreciably different from this uninfected group.[28] The yield from routine examination may be considerable; one study revealed rectal gonorrhea in 14 of 307 men (4.5 percent) and 62 of 307 women (20.1 percent) who were routinely examined.[29] Although contamination from the vagina may produce a considerable proportion of rectal gonorrhea in women, Pariser[30] found that 75 percent of women with a positive rectal culture admitted some form of penoanal contact. Of those with a positive rectal culture, 20 percent had negative cervical tests.

Anal warts suggest anal intercourse. Trauma and increased moisture may contribute to the infection.

Significance of Infection Sites

An appreciation of the common sites of infection is important for two reasons. First, infections in most of these sites (*e.g.*, cervix, rectum, pharynx) are usually asymptomatic. Secondly, routine testing of these sites in sexually active groups will reveal a high incidence of infection. Examination of the male contacts of women with gonorrhea is also likely to reveal many cases of asymptomatic urethritis. (Pariser[31] found 62 of 532 (11.6 percent) men to be asymptomatic.) Persistent asymptomatic infection may also occur after treatment.

Chapter Four

Prevention
and
Management
of
Unwanted Pregnancy

Unwanted pregnancy is one of the more serious social sequelae of sexual behavior. Certainly more difficulties are posed by its management than by the routine treatment of venereal disease. Consequently, one of the most important tasks of the venereologist is to ensure that all female patients have adequate contraceptive coverage. Both choice of prophylaxis and management of pregnancy when it occurs require the close cooperation of patient and clinician. While the patient may have precise expectations of management, she lacks the background to assess the techniques by which these are best achieved. The clinician, on his part, must appreciate that technical proficiency forms only a small component of effective prophylaxis. The optimum management of unwanted pregnancy depends largely on the feelings and attitudes of the mother, which will vary greatly from one individual to another.

Pregnancy Prophylaxis

Major considerations in the choice of prophylaxis include the patient's preference, reliability, age, and parity or the number of children she has had. The frequency and types of sexual behavior should be considered, and the efficacy and side effects of whatever technique is employed.

With the advent of more effective techniques, some methods advocated in the past are no longer applicable. Withdrawal, sometimes referred to as coitus interruptus, should not be advocated, since penile sensation is an inadequate index of emission of spermatozoa; furthermore, when practiced for long periods this technique may disrupt sexual harmony. Intravaginal preparations may have a limited role as an adjunct to other methods or when coitus is experienced infrequently, but these should not be considered for routine use. There has been a recent resurgence of interest in this method with an effort to develop a preparation both spermaticidal and bactericidal to venereally transmitted organisms. Many venereologists consider these efforts unwarranted, particularly since a highly effective prophylactic against both pregnancy and venereal disease (the condom) has existed for centuries.

Prophylaxis, therefore, must be selected from the rhythm method, the condom, hormonal medication, I.U.D., or sterilization.

Rhythm Method

The rhythm method has little appeal technically, but it does have a limited role for those individuals who refuse to use any other form of prophylaxis. Those who use rhythm effectively are usually mature and well-motivated and observe the restrictions zealously. The method relies on the limited period of fertilization, which is confined to 24–48 hours after ovulation. This usually occurs about 14 days before menstruation. By refraining from coitus within an arbitrary period, say one week during the estimated ovulation, pregnancy is avoided. The time of ovulation may be defined more precisely by regular temperature recordings. Twenty-four to 36 hours after ovulation, the basal temperature rises to a higher level, one that is maintained throughout the remainder of the premenstrual phase. Pregnancy rarely results from intercourse taking place more than 24 hours after this temperature rise. Spermatozoa from intercourse up to seven days preceding ovulation may remain viable and so fertilize the ovum after ovulation.

Condom

In addition to being a highly effective contraceptive, the condom affords protection against venereal disease. In the past, condoms were often made from thick rubber material that impaired penile sensation during intercourse and frequently caused vaginal irritation. In spite of the introduction of improved products having neither of these defects, prejudice against the condom persists. Certainly to be effective for either pregnancy or disease prophylaxis, the condom should be correctly worn throughout all phases of sexual activity. The condom may be ineffective if it is not applied until final intromission or if it is removed before all intimacies have ceased.

Highly effective and inexpensive, the condom is the prophylactic of choice when intravaginal coitus occurs infrequently.

Hormonal Methods

Hormonal methods utilize estrogens and progestogens to suppress ovulation. These hormones also inhibit the normal maturation of the endometrium and reduce the permeability of the cervical mucous. Whereas sequential administration of estrogen and progestin may be satisfactory for some individuals, a low-dose (with 50 mcg or less of estrogen) combination preparation provides the most satisfactory form for general use.

Hormonal contraception is theoretically the most effective method available of preventing pregnancy. The maximum true failure rates are 0.07 pregnancies per 100 women years for combined preparations, 0.34 for sequential contraceptives, and 2.3 for continuous oral progestogen.[2] Because hormonal contraception is not properly used, it frequently has a higher pregnancy rate than the intrauterine device.

Hormonal methods are contraindicated in patients who have

1. a history of thromboembolic disease,
2. impaired liver function or recent jaundice,
3. suspected estrogen-influenced neoplasia,
4. undiagnosed abnormal genital bleeding (including amenorrhea),
5. serious systemic illness, including hypertension, insulin-dependent diabetes, and conditions predisposing to edema.

Consequently, hormonal contraception should be preceded by a complete history and physical examination and a Papanicolaou smear. The patient should be reviewed annually. It is unwise to prescribe oral contraceptives to women who are unreliable or experience vaginal coitus infrequently. The relatively high cost is a further disadvantage of this method.

The defects of patient unreliability and cost may be countered by using an injectable preparation (*e.g.*, medroxyprogesterone acetate) which provides highly effective protection for 3–6 months. Because there may be a long delay in the reestablishment of normal ovulatory pattern after discontinuance, this preparation is contraindicated for nulliparous patients.

Intrauterine Devices (IUD)

Intrauterine devices are less effective in preventing pregnancy than hormonal contraceptives, but their users usually have a lower overall pregnancy rate because the pill is frequently not administered properly or is discontinued. Pregnancy occasionally occurs with the I.U.D. *in situ*, and the I.U.D. may be expelled without patient awareness. Menorrhagia and dysmenorrhea, the most common complications, usually subside after several menstrual periods. Major advantages over hormonal contraceptives include lower cost, greater use effectiveness, and none of the side effects from long-term exogenous hormones.

The IUD is more difficult to insert in nulliparous patients who have a higher expulsion rate than parous patients. Because of this, for reliable nulliparous patients the pill is probably the prophylactic of choice. The IUD is not necessarily contraindicated in the nulliparous patient, and it is becoming more widely used in adolescent programs. The Dalkon shield and Copper-T have been used for these patients, but paracervical anesthesia is occasionally necessary for insertion.

Insertion is contraindicated during active pelvic inflammatory disease, in pregnancy, or in the presence of congenital malformations, large fibroids, or other causes of gross deformity of the uterine cavity. Insertion is easiest during menstruation or in the immediate postpartum period.

Sterilization

Although this procedure can be reversed in some cases, it is best regarded as irreversible by the patient who is deciding upon its use. Consequently, it should be reserved for those individuals who no longer wish to reproduce either because of existing children or because of factors that are unlikely to alter during their reproductive life. Partners of a stable relationship have a choice of male or female sterilization. Physically, male sterilization is favored by the simplicity and safety of the operation, which may be performed under local anesthetic or on an outpatient basis. Female sterilization, although more complicated, is favored by clearer indications in some cases.

Psychological factors are important both in deciding on sterilization and in handling the sequelae following the operation. Detailed consultation with both partners is a prerequisite for this operation which is contraindicated if it is being used for secondary purposes or is likely to impair the sociosexual relationship between the two partners. Both partners should understand the full implications of the operation (on the assumption that it is irreversible) and the potential prophylactic limitations.

The clearest indications for tubal ligation are provided by obstetric conditions. When the dangers from further pregnancy outweigh any desire for further children, sterilization is clearly indicated. Multiparity is a relative indication and must be assessed in conjunction with age, socioeconomic status, and health of the patient. In some communities, tubal ligation is a desirable component of cesarean section. In areas of greater surgical proficiency, several cesarean sections may be performed without appreciable risk for future pregnancies. Women under 30 years of age should be sterilized only on unequivocal medical, psychiatric, or genetic grounds, or in exceptional social circumstances.

Ultimate satisfaction with tubal ligation is influenced by the stability of the marital relationship, psychiatric adjustment, and the success of the operation.

Management of Unwanted Pregnancy

Unwanted pregnacy may either be terminated or allowed to run its course. In the latter case, the mother has the choice of keeping her child or relinquishing its care to the state. The suitability of these alternatives varies greatly from one individual to another and is especially influenced by the marital status of the mother. It is rarely desirable for an unmarried mother to keep her unwanted child. Of course, some single women deliberately become pregnant in order to have a child of their own, but these pregnancies are not unwanted and are outside the scope of this discussion.

The management of unwanted pregnancy hinges on the availability of induced abortion. Until recently, most communities have harbored an emotional antagonism to this operation. Opposition to abortion *per se* centers largely on the right to life of the fetus; the operation is usually equated with murder, which is, of course, a legal term rather than a scientific one. Many physicians consider that each case should be considered individually, however, so that undesirable sequelae to the mother and society will be minimized. In some circumstances, the refusal to perform an abortion may render the physician liable to ethical or legal condemnation if such refusal directly contributes to the death of a pregnant woman. The question resolves, therefore, into a consideration of those indications for which termination is an acceptable solution.

Although physical indications generally have been considered medically respectable and while psychiatric ones have been granted grudging acceptance, there has often been reluctance to accept abortion on social grounds. In fact, both medical and psychiatric indications for termination occur infrequently. In the past, these types of indications have been used as scapegoats to allow operations on social grounds. The view that abortion can be justified on psychiatric grounds but never on purely sociological ones indicates a naive concept of the interaction of individual and environment. Such a view is characteristic of physicians who are disease-oriented but rarely have much concern for the needs of their patients. To many present-day physicians, the patients' chief role is to convey disease to the consulting room where it can be examined and dispatched with scientific expertise. While delineation of medical, psychiatric, or sociological factors may be convenient for the legislator or researcher, these are of no interest to the patient who merely recognizes that she has a complex problem for which she seeks a satisfactory solution.

The management of unwanted pregnancy, therefore, involves much more than consideration of medical indications and allowance of one of three treatment schedules. The existence of unwanted pregnancy indicates defective past management. The final solution can not be the optimal one—it will merely be the least harmful alternative. Furthermore, the total social situation of the mother and her future sexual adjustment must be prime considerations in management. The woman with unwanted pregnancy is frequently anxious and depressed. She sees termination as the perfect solution to her mental torment and intolerable life situation. The real cause of her disturbance may be her total social setting, which she is incapable of modifying. When she is offered guidance and given hope for future adjustment, the desire for termination becomes less pressing. This is especially true with many married mothers who are quite prepared to have one more child if they know it will be the last but are disturbed by the prospect of their current episode being repeated many times in the future.

One solution to unwanted pregnancy is to provide abortion to all women requesting it. The number of abortions should be restricted for several reasons. For many individuals, the risks of abortion, even when performed by experts, are greater than those of alternative contraceptive measures. Secondly, compared with prophylactic measures, abortions are demanding on hospital and medical resources. Finally, most physicians and paramedical staff consider abortion among their less pleasant duties. While many are prepared to endure this unpleasantness if it is essential for the well-being of the mother, they prefer other alternatives. For these reasons, abortion must be decided on an individual basis against the background of the relative risks involved in continuation and termination of pregnancy.

Complications of Unwanted Pregnancy

The complications of unwanted pregnancy will be borne in varying degrees by mother, child, and society. The mother may face a damaged career, social rebuke, or severe economic hardship. Depression and severe anxiety are the most common psychological responses to these prospects. Suicide may even be seen as one alternative. There is no evidence, however, that women with unwanted pregnancy make a disproportionate contribution to the suicide rate.

Since 25–50 percent of the single women who are denied legal abortion will persist in seeking abortion until they obtain it, whether legally or illegally, a proportion of these women will have illegal abortions at a more advanced stage of pregnancy, with a consequent dramatic increase in the risk of complications.

Although liberal abortion laws will save the lives of some women and will decrease morbidity for many others, their impact on criminal abortion is uncertain. The assumption that abortion on demand will eliminate criminal abortion is not substantiated by the existing evidence.

The impact on the unwanted child depends largely on his placement. Adoption is associated with the most favorable outcome. These children probably fare at least as well as the remainder of the populace. Race, physical handicap, or other defects may militate against adoption. These individuals face institutionalization with its dismal prognosis. Those children who remain with an unmarried mother may encounter problems of similar magnitude. Lack of a father demands compensatory love and support from the mother, but these women often provide less than average affection and care for their offspring. A similar social environment may be encountered by children in very large families when the limited parental support (material and emotional) is exhausted by other siblings. In situations of diminished parental contact, the child's maladjustment is manifested as increased antisocial behavior and delinquency.

Techniques for Termination

The risks of termination are determined largely by the stage of pregnancy and the competence of the operator. When practiced as an epidemiologic measure, abortion should be performed only by a specialized gynecologist and be restricted to pregnancies of less than twelve weeks, and preferably less than ten weeks duration.

The recommended method is suction evacuation performed under local anesthesia in a fully equipped operating theatre at the clinic. After four hours of bed rest, the patient is allowed to leave, with a review scheduled in four days. The operating clinic should be within twenty minutes traveling time of a full surgical facility that may be utilized for the rare postoperative emergencies that may arise.

Dilatation and curettage, an alternative to suction, complicates over-all management, since general anesthesia and overnight hospitalization are desirable for this procedure.

Complications of Termination

Complications may be physical or psychological. The major physical complications—sepsis, hemorrhage, or their manifestations—are minimal when abortion is performed before ten weeks by an experienced specialist.

Psychological complications may be immediate or remote and are more nebulous than the physical sequelae. Guilt, self-reproach, and regret may be experienced by some women, but these symptoms are rarely severe. Reservations tend to be more common among married women who are aborted for medical, rather than for social reasons. Psychological complications, as influenced both by the attitudes of society and the adequacy of pre- and post-termination counseling, will probably decline in incidence in the future.

Accumulated experience in the United States has enabled an objective assessment of the risks associated with termination.[3] These statistics, summarized in Table 4-1, demonstrate the dramatic increase in complications and maternal mortality with an increase in the duration of pregnancy. Concurrent sterilization and preexisting medical problems (e.g., diabetes, heart disease, or gynecological problems) also increase the risk of complications. Early abortion is associated with fewer psychiatric complications and lower maternal mortality than uninterrupted pregnancy.

For comparison with the mortality figures of early termination, the surgical removal of tonsils and adenoids had a mortality risk of 5: 100,000 operations in the United States in 1969.

Assessment of Unwanted Pregnancy

In assessing the optimum management for each individual situation, the following factors should be considered.

The patient's true feelings towards termination. Often the patient requests an abortion because she thinks it is the normal thing to do, or because of pressures from husband or family. Termination should not be considered unless the patient is an enthusiastic proponent of the operation on her own initiative.

TABLE 4-1 SEQUELAE OF ABORTION IN THE UNITED STATES[3]

Medical Complications (per 100 abortions)

	First Trimester	Second Trimester
Not Sterilized Concurrently		
No other medical problems	0.6	2.1
Other medical problems	2.0	6.7
Concurrent Sterilization		
No other medical problems	7.2	8.0
Other medical problems	17	17

Psychological Complications

Post abortion psychosis (per 1000)	0.2–0.4
Post pregnancy psychosis (per 1000)	1–2

Maternal Mortality (per 100,000)

Legal Abortion	
Under 8 weeks	0.5
9–10 weeks	1.7
11–12 weeks	4.2
16–20 weeks	Over 17
Hysterotomy or hysterectomy techniques	61.3
Pregnancy	
Natural delivery	14
Cesarean section	111

The attitudes of the child's father.   Financial and emotional support from the father are critical. If the patient continues to associate with the child's father, antagonism or even ambivalence on his part is likely to produce conflicts and unhappiness for both the mother and child. If social connections with the father have been severed, support from some other source is essential.

The attitudes and support available from the patient's parents, family doctor, and peers.   Continuing financial and emotional support is essential for the unmarried mother. In the absence of a husband, this must be provided by some other intimate associate. A father-figure is also important for healthy psychosocial development of the child.

Previous pregnancies and their outcome.   These provide some indication of the physical or psychological sequelae likely from continuation. The number of existing children and their ages influence the financial and emotional burden on the mother but may also indicate a source of some support.

The age, maturity, socioeconomic status, marital status, personality and psychological stability of the patient.   All these factors give an indication of the patient's ability to cope with continuation or termination of pregnancy.

The impact of continuation or termination on the patient's profession or career. Even where this factor is not critical for financial support, sacrifice by the mother may be reflected in hostility to the child.

The reason for the unwanted pregnancy and whether it is likely to recur. Repeated abortion is an unsatisfactory method of coping with recurrent unwanted pregnancy. If recurrence is likely, some permanent form of prophylaxis should be provided.

Physical illness of the patient. Physical illness is rarely severe enough to prevent either safe termination or continuation of pregnancy, but it may be critical in determining the patient's ability to provide sole support over a long period for her child.

The patient's religious convictions. The patient should be aware of the attitudes and laws of the religious organizations with which she is affiliated and should understand the impact of her proposed actions on this affiliation. By contrast, the physician should not be influenced by his own religious convictions but should advise solely on medicosocial grounds—the field of expertise in which he is being consulted.

Regardless of any decision about termination, adequate prophylaxis and support for the future must be provided to ensure that unwanted pregnancy does not recur.

Bibliography

Baird D: Sterilization and therapeutic abortion in Aberdeen, Br J Psychiatry 113: 703, 1967

Barglow P, Klass D: Psychiatric aspects of contraceptive utilization, Am J Obstet Gynecol 114: 93, 1972

Baudry F, Wiener A: The pregnant patient in conflict about abortion: a challenge for the obstetrician, Am J Obstet Gynecol 119: 705, 1974

Blacker CP, Peel JM: Sterilization of women, Br Med J 1:566, 1969

Borland BL: Behavioral factors in non-coital methods of contraception: a review, Soc Sci Med 6: 163, 1972

Edelman DA, Brenner WE, Berger GS: The effectiveness and complications of abortion by dilatation and vacuum aspiration versus dilatation and rigid metal curettage, Am J Obstet Gynecol 19: 473, 1974

Elstein M: The present status of contraception, Practitioner 208: 485, 1972

Forsmann, H, Thuwe I: One hundred and twenty children born after application for therapeutic abortion was refused: their mental health, social adjustment and educational level up to the age of 21, Acta Psychiatr Scand 42: 71, 1966

Hanley HG: Vasectomy for voluntary male sterilization, Lancet 2: 207, 1968

Helper MM, Cohen RL, Beitenman ET, Eaton LF: Life events and acceptance of pregnancy, J Psychosom Res, 30: 183, 1968

Hook K: Refused abortion: a follow up study of 249 women whose applications were refused by the national board of health in Sweden, Acta Psychiatr Scand [Suppl.] 168, 1963

Kerslake D, Casey D: Abortion induced by means of the uterine aspirator, Obstet Gynecol, 30: 35, 1967

Marinoff SC: Contraception in adolescents, Pediatr Clin North Am 19: 811, 1972

Rodger TF: Attitudes toward abortion, Am J Psychiatry 125: 116, 1968

Simon NM, Senturia AG: Psychiatric sequelae of abortion, Arch Gen Psychiatry 15: 378, 1966

Swyer GI: Advances in hormonal contraception, Practitioner 211: 535, 1973

Tredgold RF: Psychiatric indications for termination of pregnancy, Lancet, 2: 1251, 1964

White RB: Induced abortions—a survey of their psychiatric implications, complications and indications, Tex Rep Biol Med 24: 531, 1966

Chapter Five

Promiscuity
and
Prostitution

Promiscuity

Promiscuity is intimate sexual behavior on the basis of casual association. This indulgence in intimate behavior in an indiscriminate manner in the absence of an established social relationship almost inevitably ensures that promiscuous individuals will have a large number of sexual partners. This is the facet of promiscuity relevant to venereal disease. Prostitution is an obvious example of promiscuity on a commercial basis, but promiscuity for pleasure is more common in modern Western society. This latter phenomenon exists as two distinct entities: transient promiscuity and habitual promiscuity.

Transient Promiscuity

Transient promiscuity is an adaptive process, although a morally unsatisfactory one, of the socially immature. Its incidence is influenced by the attitudes and structure of society, but it is practiced by essentially normal responsible individuals as part of their social development. In his search for a happy and satisfying relationship, the promiscuous individual chooses a partner casually but discards her when the relationship does not fulfill his expectations. In the normal individual this is an adaptive process, however. With subsequent partners he is more discriminating. The unions become progressively more stable until eventually he abandons his promiscuous pattern and establishes a permanent relationship.

During the adjustment period venereal disease, unwanted pregnancy, and psychological distress may occur. The individual usually feels a sense of responsibility when these sequelae occur in his partner. He usually cooperates willingly with those who endeavor to minimize the impact of his actions both at a personal and a community level. He learns from his mistakes, and, following appropriate advice and support, his problems rarely recur. The hardships arising from such sequelae are often unnecessarily aggravated by an intolerant society. Family rejection of the unmarried mother, moralizing, begrudging medical counsel, and social persecution of the venereally infected may convert an unfortunate predicament into a socially and psychologically disastrous one.

Figure 5-1 demonstrates the way in which transient promiscuity is inextricably related to other processes of sexual adjustment. It shows how the relative contribution of any institution or process is determined solely by the overall attitudes and structure of society. A direct assault on any component, while altering the form it takes, will have no influence on its overall contribution. Legal sanctions against prostitution, for example, will produce an increase in clandestine prostitution but will not alter the contribution of prostitution to sexual outlet. In a permissive society where transient promiscuous relationships are readily available, prostitution will decline because of reduced demand. The contribution of masturbation will be determined largely by the availability of heterosexual or homosexual partners; attitudes or sanctions against masturbation merely influence the furtiveness with which it is practiced. The contribution of marriage to sexual outlet is influenced by societal structure and attitudes and socioeconomic factors. Altering the ease of divorce has no influence on its overall contribution; it merely determines the proportion of legal marriages which serve a meaningful function.

Habitual Promiscuity

> Habitually promiscuous individuals never reach full sexual maturity, each of their numerous sexual affairs has a playful character and resembles masturbatory gratification more than a mature union, the multiplicity of their affairs points to search for the unobtainable.[1]

Habitual promiscuity is a pathologic process closely associated

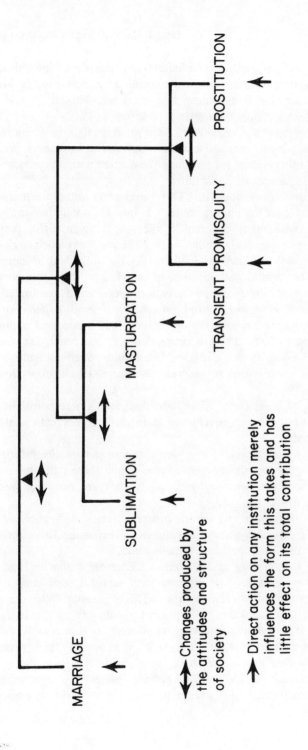

MARRIAGE

SUBLIMATION

MASTURBATION

TRANSIENT PROMISCUITY

PROSTITUTION

↕ Changes produced by the attitudes and structure of society

→ Direct action on any institution merely influences the form this takes and has little effect on its total contribution

FIGURE 5–1 THE BALANCE OF SEXUAL OUTPUT IN A SOCIETY

with the sociopathic personality. The habitually promiscuous individual attempts to alleviate by sexual excess the social deficiencies due to his personality disorder. He is a menace to society and himself.

This condition includes a number of features.

Impulsive, irresponsible behavior. The individual is quite indiscriminate. He may have intercourse with a partner he has never previously met. His sole concern is immediate satisfaction without consideration of the consequences of his actions.

The behavior is non-adaptive. This behavior is initially a manifestation of a search for the unobtainable. The individual may habitually have intercourse with many different partners in a given night. Any satisfaction is purely physical. Rather than enhancing any social relationship, his behavior alienates his partners. As the individual becomes addicted to this behavioral pattern, orgasm becomes the sole goal; but the satisfaction is short-lived, and so the pattern recurs and is reinforced.

Marked inability to profit from mistakes and modify behavior. Venereal disease may be acquired 5 or 10 times but is accepted philosophically as a part of life. There is no tendency to use prophylaxis or alter behavior, for this is not considered necessary. Such individuals, therefore, make a contribution to venereal disease out of all proportion to their numbers.

Lack of social conscience. The individual feels no responsibility for the unwanted pregnancies, psychological distress, or venereal disease which he propagates.

There may be a marked discrepancy between personality adjustment and intelligence or manual competence. While these latter talents are frequently used to attain short-term goals, they are rarely utilized for long-term adjustment in society.

The ability to impress and exploit others. Their intelligence, natural ability, and plausible extroverted manner often make these individuals very likeable on superficial acquaintance.

Intolerance to authority and discipline. External authority is accepted only so long as it does not interfere with personal preferences.

Impaired interpersonal relationships. This deficiency follows automatically from the completely self-centered personality of the individual. After the initial good impression, the deception is inevitably unmasked. The immediate reaction of associates is hostility and anger at being duped. Often this is tempered by the facile lying and the excuses of the sociopath. As deceptions continue, however, interpersonal relationships deteriorate and eventually any good will becomes irrecoverable.

In contact with the venereologist these individuals frequently erect a facade of cooperation that is particularly dangerous, for it encourages the unwary to place undeserved trust in their obedience and reliability. In fact, they provide inadequate trace reports, are unreliable in taking medication, may continue promiscuous behavior while still infective, and often default. They are quite unreceptive to counseling of any type —they consider the blame for their situation rests entirely with society. While management of these individuals is frustrating, it will be associated with less personal and community distress if the clinician is aware of his patient's deceptive character.

While the female analogue to the habitually promiscuous male probably exists, the "very promiscuous" females seen with venereal disease more often fit a different social pattern. They contribute disproportionately to venereal disease, are unreliable, and are not particularly receptive to counseling, but for different reasons than the male. Their intelligence tends to parallel their personality and social deficiencies, and they are readily exploited by the male sociopath. Sexual behavior is used for nonsexual ends, but their goal is usually increased social acceptance rather than physical pleasure. Many probably make a genuine effort to cooperate with the clinician, but they fail because they are generally incompetent. They forget to take the pill. They forget to take medication. They cannot resist sexual relations regardless of whether they are infected, claim dyspareunia, or have any other disability.

The more intelligent promiscuous female sociopath probably tends to enter prostitution rather than be exploited without material gain. While she may still be exploited by a pimp or a madam, she is offered some psychological compensation by exploiting her clients.

Prostitution

Definition

Views on prostitution are often grossly distorted. This is because of the emotional disgust with which a large proportion of the community regard this institution and because of unwarranted generalizations and oversimplications about a most complex and diverse sociological phenomenon. Among the few valid generalizations about prostitution is its noteworthy diversity and flexibility. Any consideration of prostitution or prostitutes must carefully isolate both component sociological units and their participants, who may bear little resemblance to one another. The streetwalker, brothel whore, gangster's moll, clandestine prostitute, hetaera, and geisha span a spectrum of human types probably as wide as that encountered in all the sexual participants in any one community.

Difficulties in defining prostitution arise largely from an exclusive focus on its commercial nature. Although it is true that prostitution is fundamentally a commercial enterprise, definition on this criterion alone is not without problems. Sexual attractiveness is a valuable negotiable commodity. It is commercially exploited, at least indirectly, by a large proportion of most populations. Negotiation using sexual attractiveness is not limited to the human race, for higher mammals are also aware of its value.[2] In this respect it is not different from physical strength, intelligence, or other personal attributes that may give those well endowed in these qualities a selective advantage for material or intangible betterment. The sexually attractive woman may, purely on account of this attractiveness, enjoy an exciting social life, receive expensive gifts, and choose a marriage partner who is likely to guarantee a comfortable future either materially or psychologically. This exploitation, which is almost universal, is not consciously recognized as such by many who employ it. They would certainly abhor the suggestion that they were exploiting sex for commercial gain. Yet from a purely commercial point of view, the difference between this behavior and prostitution is merely a matter of degree.

A more definitive quality of prostitution is its lack of selectivity and emotional indifference. Providing a client has the money, he will be serviced. Since the client is probably a complete stranger and may be physically unattractive and perverted in inclinations, he is unlikely to engender any positive emotional response in his partner. More relevantly, even if these factors are not operating, it is economically expedient for the prostitute to process her clients as mechanically as possible. Hence the most appropriate definition of *prostitution* is sexual intercourse on a promiscuous and mercenary basis accompanied by emotional indifference.[3]

Although this may be the best available definition, it is in fact inadequate. With the great diversity of prostitution, emotional indifference and lack of selectivity are not inevitable concomitants. High-class prostitutes may select clients strictly with regard to their wealth and physical and behavioral characteristics. In some cases selection is certainly much stricter than some women apply in selecting a husband. Furthermore, there may be considerable emotional attachment to some clients. Still other women, who are unquestionably prostitutes practicing their trade, may not even be particularly concerned about the commercial nature of their contracts with some partners. They may decline payment or leave the amount of payment entirely to the discretion of the client, who is usually a regular customer or may for some reason have particular empathy with the prostitute. In contrast, emotional indifference, resignation, or even resentment is not an uncommon occurrence in intercourse between marital partners.

It is therefore apparent that there is no single unambiguous definition of prostitution. This is a positive rather than a negative finding, for it highlights prostitution as a component of sexual gratification. Prostitution represents a segment on a continuum of modes of sexual expression, but the actual beginning and ending of this segment is ill-defined and can only be delineated arbitrarily.

This leads to the central fact of prostitution. As a commercial enterprise, every facet of its organization including its very existence is determined either largely or entirely by customer demand. Prostitution develops in response to demand, and any interference with it must deal primarily with this demand or the outcome will be unsatisfactory. Moreover, prostitution and its manifestations are irrevocably related to promiscuity and other behavior patterns outside of prostitution. Any alteration in one kind of behavior inevitably produces a reflex change in the other.

It is appropriate therefore to consider in more detail various aspects of this demand, the flexibility of prostitution in meeting the demand, and the rational and irrational mechanisms by which societies have reacted to this institution.

Types of Prostitution

The patterns of prostitution may vary widely both between societies and within a particular society. Changes in the prevalence of prostitution, as assessed by the number of participants who are known to regulating institutions, may indicate no more than a change in this pattern. While the various forms of prostitution may be considered to have their origins in an evolutionary process,[4] each really depends on a particular type of social organization with particular standards and behavior patterns. Types of prostitution that are of waning significance in a society may readily be restored through sudden social disturbance.

Unorganized prostitution. This can be expected to arise when there is a major disturbance to the male:female sex ratio. Scheinfeld[5] suggests, "the most stable and moral community is the one where there is an almost equal number of both sexes, with just a slight excess of men." Travelers or itinerant workers will disturb this ratio and may create a demand for prostitution. In societies where promiscuous behavior is accepted and the demand is not great, transitory relationships on a noncommercial basis may cope with this demand. Where more rigid mores prevail, however, there will be fewer women prepared to indulge such liaisons, the demand will be greater, and the commercial value of the provided commodity more apparent. Paradoxically, prostitution is encouraged by rigid social standards that preclude a large proportion of the female pool from promiscuity. Such standards enhance the relative value of those few who are prepared to transgress them. Prostitution is likely to remain at a relatively unorganized stage where the number of potential clients is not great and where community development is simple, i.e., in developing countries or underprivileged areas of developed countries.

Organized prostitution.   This form of prostitution occurs in more sophisticated communities or at times when the number of potential clients and hence financial return become greater. The *streetwalker* obtains clients by openly mingling with the crowd and securing customers as the opportunity arises. She may frequent street corners as her name suggests, but bars, hotel lobbies, wharves, or other localities where there is likely to be a high proportion of potential clients, are popular haunts. Having obtained a client, the contract is concluded in a private room, hotel, mobile vehicle, or other prearranged location. The prostitute frequently works alone, but she may belong to a group managed by a pimp or to a much larger organization. Because the streetwalker is generally regarded as being of low status among prostitutes, this field is often occupied by a high proportion of women either at the beginning of their career or in its twilight when their desirability is less and they must seek whatever trade is available.

Brothel prostitution.   When the demand for commercial sex becomes very great, brothels provide one solution. This represents the mass production or factory stage of the commercial enterprise. There can be no pretense of providing quality. The sole object is to process as many clients as quickly as possible. This system flourishes during wartime or in other situations where a large number of men are separated from their womenfolk. In more stable communities, organized houses of prostitution are often restricted to certain areas, producing the redlight districts, which in the past have been a feature of so many cities. Girls are recruited to these houses by a variety of means and serve a type of apprenticeship in adjusting to the requirements of their trade.

With the increasing complexity of the institution, exploitation of the prostitute becomes a significant feature. As in many other large organizations, the worker at the lowest level may receive a trifling proportion of the profit from the industry. The madam who manages the house often maintains firm control over the total life of her charges and deducts a high percentage of the girl's earnings for expenses. In turn, a disproportionate share of the profits may be earmarked for the controllers of the house and for police protection. By this means a large proportion of the earnings of prostitution is distributed to ostensibly respectable citizens—including business leaders, politicians, and the police. In other instances the earnings pass to more obviously criminal syndicates.

In Eastern countries, the "bar" is a variation on this class of prostitution. The prostitute works ostensibly as a hostess, receiving a commission for the drinks she induces customers to buy. A customer may make an appointment for intercourse after the girl has ceased her bar duties. Alternatively, he may buy her out of the bar, paying the madam a sum equivalent to her earnings for the remainder of the day. Dance halls and a number of other institutions operate on the same principle. Some girls in these establishments will not have intercourse with customers. This is not due to moral reasons nor does it exclude them from prostitution—the prime motive is monetary. The attractive sought-after girl may receive far greater financial return from her bar commission than from resorting to intercourse. To achieve this it is necessary to provide an array of sexual stimulation to her customers, including masturbation to orgasm and fellatio.

Clandestine prostitution. With changes in societal reaction and the demands of a new type of client, clandestine prostitution rises to increased prominence. The *call girl* and the *high-class independent professional prostitute* are the two most obvious examples of this group. They aim at providing a higher quality performance for a more selected clientele.

This type of prostitute has greater status. This status "is based on her attractiveness, financial standing, political connections, dress, apartment, manners and the state in which she keeps her 'old man' or pimp."[6] Greenwald mentions various types of prostitute which gives some appreciation of the diversity, even in one category, of this profession. The party girl has only one date an evening, never explicitly mentions a fee, and may restrict her clients to men with some appeal. The hustler or hooker operates on an appointment basis. The kept woman maintains a relationship with one man at a time in return for financial security while their arrangement is in existence.

The call girl makes contact with her clients by telephone, either directly or more commonly *via* an answering service. Clients are obtained by exchange with other prostitutes, recommendations from previous clients, or through a variety of procurers—including taxi drivers, desk clerks, and convention organizers. The contact is conducted preferably in the client's home or hotel room, but sometimes the call girl must use an apartment of her own. The call girls interviewed by Greenwald "earned in the neighborhood of twenty thousand dollars a year." The charge for each session was usually twenty to a hundred dollars but occasionally more. As one call girl commented, "A man spending this amount of money expects deception and romance, as well as the orgasm."

The independent professional prostitute caters to a still more selective clientele and has less contact with the rest of the prostitute world. She has her own apartment in which she conducts her business. She frequently has another job, however, and uses prostitution to supplement her earnings.

Societal Involvement

Prostitution is condemned because it is an affront to the morals of society. Society expects sex to be confined to stable social relationships where procreation is its goal. Instead, in prostitution, one partner uses sex for money and the other for pleasure.

Prostitution may gain increased acceptance in a number of ways: 1) if there is some degree of discrimination in selecting clients; 2) if the proceeds of prostitution are used for a socially desirable purpose; 3) if the purely commercial nature of the act is disguised in any way.[7]

Examples of this elevation in esteem are apparent both throughout history and at the present time. The hetaerae of Greece, by adding cultural companionship to sexual gratification, enjoyed elevated status over other prostitutes. In Japan, the *joro* in the brothels, the *jogoku* on the streets, and the geisha, or entertainers, occupy distinctly separate strata of esteem.

The clandestine prostitute disguises her prostitution behind a facade of respectability. By being selective, providing entertainment, and receiving payment in a covert manner, the mercenary nature of her sex is attenuated. Concurrent employment in a respectable occupation and residence in a high-class area fosters the self-deception that she is not a prostitute. Society, in turn, respects the fact that she does not flaunt her prostitution.

The temple prostitution of India can be accepted because the proceeds benefit the temple, and the sexual act can be rationalized as an act of worship.

Regulation of Prostitution

In practice, society is faced with two approaches to the control of prostitution—toleration or suppression.[8] In view of the moralistic standards of society, full acceptance is not considered a practical possibility.

Limited toleration assumes that prostitution is inevitable but that its manifestations must be curbed in some way. When prostitution has been tolerated in a limited manner, three classic regulation methods have emerged. The first of these is regulation by inscription in which registration of prostitutes is compulsory. Prostitutes have regular health checks for venereal or other disease.

Registration has been opposed on the grounds that it infringes the civil rights of the individual and is contrary to modern conceptions of humanity (Article 6 of the United Nations Resolution on Prostitution, 1950). It effectively labels a woman and may make it more difficult for her to become reestablished in a respectable occupation.[9] Furthermore, registration will be notoriously incomplete in that a large proportion of clandestine prostitutes and those with influence remain unregistered.[10]

Compulsory medical examination of prostitutes has proven valueless in controlling venereal disease. Such examinations may be harmful, in fact, because spuriously favorable results provide a false sense of security both to clients and controllers. They may also provoke hostility and consequent decreased cooperation from the prostitutes themselves.

Willcox[11] quotes several examples of the extremely low returns that may result from compulsory examination. In one study of three thousand Paris prostitutes in 1948, 83,400 examinations yielded 229 cases of venereal disease (0.27 percent). In another study, 294 cases were obtained from 98,992 examinations (0.30 percent). Another provided 27 cases from 3,794 examinations (0.71 percent). Contrarily, inadequate diagnostic criteria may reverse these findings by showing inflated yields.

Bettley[12] has given an account of a fully organized brothel which was established in an overseas country strictly for the use of military personnel. This was controlled by military police and was stocked with 30–40 prostitutes of various races aged 18 to 40. Each woman averaged 30 clients a day. The prostitutes were examined by a civilian doctor prior to employment and at weekly intervals. Prophylactics were provided and preventive ablution was utilized after intercourse. The VD rate was 0.31/1000 for those using prophylaxis and 0.72/1000 for those who did not.

In contrast, legalized prostitution for American armed forces in Italy proved less successful.[13] Prostitutes were registered with the police and the houses inspected. Prophylaxis was provided and prostitutes were examined every second day. Nevertheless, over 80 percent of new infections among troops were acquired in licenced houses. This was not surprising, for infected women were allowed to continue working. Lentino explained the inadequacy of regular examination by saying, "Medical inspection of prostitutes, even when performed with the utmost scrupulousness and honesty cannot determine with even reasonable accuracy the infectivity of a prostitute."

In World War I the French government had an elaborate system of control. American army medical officers concluded that it was ineffectual and dangerous, because it created a false sense of security.[14] Dudley[15] agrees that licenced houses under medical supervision have proved more a menace than a safeguard. This same sentiment is supported by Bullough[16] with relation to prostitution in the United States: "Medically, the belief that a superficial fortnightly examination of the registered women would protect her patrons from venereal infection was found to be illusory; in fact, instead of curtailing infection such examination encouraged a false feeling of safety on the part of the prostitutes' customers."

In Cairo in World War II over 90 percent of the prostitutes in the tolerated or "clean" brothels and over 70 percent of streetwalkers were infected.[17] In India, despite complex organization and examination of prostitutes employed by the army, the VD rate rose from 166.7/1000 in 1873 to 342.7/1000 in 1885.[18]

The weakness of any system of regulation is the almost inevitable corruption of both civilian and military controllers. Greenberg[19] describes the problem confronting American forces as "a disinclination to suppress prostitution on the part of most civil authorities and actual involvement by some." Lees,[20] observing the same obstruction to British policies, said that "in Greece it was almost impossible to enforce the policy, because the Government sponsored the brothel system." This corruption was countered in Hamburg by the appointment of 16 "morality police," all of whom were married and over 35. The brothels were well organized, with prophylactic facilities and twice-weekly medical examinations, but venereal disease remained uncontrolled.[21]

Another means of expressing limited toleration is regulation by licencing. Houses of prostitution may be licenced in the same way as liquor houses are licenced. The aim in both cases is the same—to confine the sale of the commodity to a limited number of establishments which are subject to periodic surveillance.

Finally, regulation by segregation may be an alternative. By confining prostitution to certain localities it is kept from the public eye. It is then easier for the populace to rationalize that the practice does not exist. This policy gives rise to the red-light districts and the famous streets that have been a feature of many cities in the past. These are now less common because of the emergence of other forms of prostitution.[22]

Repression, Suppression or Abolition of Prostitution

The suppression of prostitution may involve keeping women off the streets, passing or enforcing measures against soliciting, or an effort to eliminate the prostitute completely.

In 1254, Louis IX of France attempted to eliminate prostitution by deporting all prostitutes and punishing those associated with the trade. All these measures failed completely. Subsequent efforts over the centuries to eliminate prostitution have been no more successful.[23]

Suppression may at least confer some short-term benefits. In 1941 when prostitution was flourishing in El Paso, Texas, the nearby army VD rate was 83/1000, 78 percent of which was acquired in brothels. When prostitution was repressed in 1942, the VD rate fell, and 47.5 percent of infections were traced to pickups. Similarly, the abolition of prostitution in Hawaii in 1944 was followed by a drop in both military and civilian VD rates.[24] The abolition of prostitution in France in 1946 also produced a decrease in venereal disease.[25]

In World War II, British policy in Germany was to place brothels out of bounds for troops.[26] Since that time American forces have adopted a similar policy in the Far East.[27] In Cairo, this approach caused a marked reduction in the VD rate within two weeks; in six months the rate was halved.[28]

When such measures have been employed, however, prostitution has inevitably demonstrated its versatility. New patterns of the profession have emerged. An environment of suppression is the ideal medium in which vice flourishes and exploitation of the prostitute reaches its height. In such a situation the law-enforcing authority, whether military or civil police, is placed in a strong position to profit illicitly from prostitution. Rarely does this opportunity pass unheeded. There are police forces which maintain their integrity against all other temptations, but there are few that have untarnished reputations following significant encounters with prostitution.[29] This view is quoted by Henriques.[30]

"The police are the brothel keeper's best friends. . . . They keep things snug. And the brothel keepers are the police's best friends, 'cos they pay them." In nineteenth-century London this remuneration might have been $3 for a small house or up to $500 a year for larger houses, plus access to the inmates.

Exploitation of the Prostitute

The prostitute is widely exploited by a large proportion of any community in which she operates. The earnings of prostitution are distributed widely among the rest of the community. The madam, the pimp, and a host of procurers—taxi drivers, desk clerks, and others—may extract more than half of her earnings directly. The police, criminal syndicates, lawyers, judges, abortionists, and other medical practitioners may all receive substantial sums to maintain the prostitute in effective working condition. Hotels, landlords, and an array of entrepreneurs also profit from prostitution.

In fact, the prostitute is exploited by society itself. The prostitute herself is made the scapegoat for prostitution, an institution that is made necessary solely by other members of society. Her needs are ignored and any superficial interest in her welfare is purely for the benefit of her customers. In terms of society's attitude to the prostitute, her moral worth and the fact that she may in turn exploit her customers toward whom she is often contemptuous, are irrelevant. The control of any social group for a protracted period of time requires the cooperation of that group. Prostitutes are no exception. It would appear that a prerequisite for better control of the problems associated with prostitution is the acceptance of the prostitute as a person and the provision of social and medical help for her own rather than others' benefit.

Characteristics of Prostitutes

Many reports about prostitutes are misleading because of a heavy bias in sampling. This may occur if the sample is very small or if certain characteristics are linked directly to the method of sampling. It is common practice, for example, to study prostitutes who have been arrested by the police or have been referred for medical assessment.[31] While this is convenient, it is unlikely that the findings bear close resemblance to those for prostitutes in general. Due to the diversity among prostitutes, generalizations on their characters are strictly limited, but there are some features that are applicable to a large proportion of the profession.

In terms of sexuality the prostitute probably differs little from the rest of the populace. She is frigid with her clients and may despise them, but she is mostly capable of enjoying normal sexual relations in other circumstances. To a considerable extent her success depends on how well she can deceive her client regarding her own emotions, "while lavishing smiles on their customers, [she] thoroughly detested them."[32]

> Feigning sexual pleasure in the embrace of a paunchy perspiring police captain is about as liberating as a hair shirt. "These guys pant and moan and I've got to pant and moan," says Lois. "They think they're giving you such a thrill. If they only knew. I could be shampooing my hair while they're working their wonders on me."[33]

Certainly hypersexuality is rare among prostitutes. This quality in no way benefits, and may hinder them in their occupation—"nymphomaniacs are rare among prostitutes."[34]

The fundamental characteristic of prostitutes is the great importance they place on material wealth in preference to moral or spiritual values. While this trait may correlate with low intellect, limited education, or a squalid upbringing, it occurs in all educational and social classes. It predisposes not only to prostitution but also to other endeavors with a mercenary bias. The prostitute tends to focus on the present with little thought for the future, a tendency which limits her motivation to change her profession. She prefers to spend her money rather than to save it and has great delight in her material possessions.

A good deal has been written about the mentality of prostitutes, much of it with little foundation. One might expect that prostitution might have more than its share of the intellectually retarded, if only due to the areas from which it draws its recruits. This fact has, however, been exaggerated by the studies of prostitutes who might be expected to have lower intelligence than the rest of their profession, e.g., those caught by the police or found in mental institutions. As Hijmans[35] writes, "It has become apparent that very many of the regular prostitutes, well known to the police in a number of countries are mentally deficient," but the key phrase relating to mental deficiency is "well known to the police" and not "regular prostitutes" as the writer implies. The statement that "the intellectual level of prostitutes is not high, for they hail from circles of low intellectual development" is more balanced. It would be fairer still if its application to "some prostitutes" were stressed. Certainly the implications of Schwarz's comment, "careful investigations have proved that the genuine prostitute is not only morally but also mentally defective"[36] must be rejected. There is ample evidence from knowledge of the existence of intelligent prostitutes to prove this statement false. Moreover, no such "careful investigations" are available, since the great majority of intelligent and successful prostitutes would not submit themselves to study, unless perhaps they were highly paid for so doing. Scheinfeld[37] concluded that prostitutes probably have intelligence similar to that of the average population. Polly Adler[38] considers "most of at least average intelligence." Although her impartiality may be disputed, she has at least had significantly more firsthand experience than some other writers on the subject.

In the absence of any more definite evidence it is probable that prostitutes tend to have lower intelligence than the average population (there is little doubt that the same applies to many groups which are considered quite normal for whom the issue of intelligence is never raised), but this is of limited sociological significance. Certainly the view that prostitutes as a class are so mentally defective as to require legal protection from their customers cannot be substantiated.

In view of the unacceptability of prostitution by society, Jackman and others[39] suggest "that these women develop a set of beliefs which counteract the social anathema attached to their way of life." Their rationalization is achieved both by denigrating others and by disputing the degree of society's disapproval. They consider that many women, including wives, use sex for ulterior purposes. They themselves are merely less hypocritical by doing so openly. They argue that there is always a demand for prostitutes, and they are only providing a service to society by meeting this demand. Although society may openly condemn them, it really welcomes the existence of prostitution as a means of protecting its other institutions.

Clients of Prostitutes

Some men will patronize a prostitute under certain environmental conditions but not others; some will resort to prostitutes for certain sexual pleasures but not others; a few individuals rely on prostitutes for most of their sexual outlet most of the time.

Henriques[40] has formulated a classification of the contemporary clientele of the prostitute.

Sado-masochistic perverts. Many men are unwilling to indulge perverse cravings or abnormal ventures into eroticism with wives or close acquaintances. There will always be some prostitutes who if provided with sufficient monetary return will satisfy virtually any experience that men can envisage, regardless of the depravity involved.[41] One study cited by Henriques[42] suggested that prostitutes' clients were divided as follows: 29 percent free of any perversion, 19 percent masochists, 14 percent fetishists, 11 percent voyeurs, 10 percent masochists with homosexual tendencies, 9 percent sadists, and 9 percent pornolists. Fellatio is popular among some clients and is reported to be currently common in France where it can be performed quickly in the back seat of a car. Greenwald[43] suggests that 75 percent–90 percent of customers of call girls wish to have orogenital acts. A predilection for old whores has been reported from New York. This may represent a desire for self-degradation by the clients.[44]

Flagellation and the provision of very young girls were practices attracting a large clientele in nineteenth-century English brothels.[45] Adler[46] comments, from American experience, "Whorehouses always draw twisted people who are unable to satisfy their desires normally."

Associated with occupation. Sailors, soldiers, and travelers may frequently be in a position where prostitutes are the only females to whom they have access in their brief contact with a community.

The functionally impotent. Because of upbringing or psychological problems, an individual may be impotent with a close acquaintance but function normally with a prostitute.[47]

The malformed, diseased, and lonely. Some men may be so physically handicapped, markedly unattractive, or tethered by defective personality that they despair of success with respectable women. In all environments loneliness is a potent motivation. Some men may linger with a prostitute for her company rather than for any sexual stimulation. "In the end one has to be brutal to remind them of what they are and where they are, and that their time is up."[48] Some individuals are virtually driven to prostitution by the prejudices of society. The immigrant may face a virtual taboo on sexual relations with the women of his adopted society and consequently will patronize the prostitute.[49]

The adolescent. This clientele is related to the Christian ideal of chastity outside marriage. With delayed marriage, the adolescent's sexual outlet depends on prostitution or promiscuity for pleasure. The distribution between these two sources will depend on the permissiveness of society.

The normal man. The normal man may have intercourse with a prostitute as the result of a fortuitous encounter, possibly in a moment of weakness or when influenced by peers or alcohol. Clinard[50] has listed some logical reasons why a man may choose a prostitute for sexual relations. 1) The prostitute is cheaper than the respectable woman. For the man who is only interested in sex, it is uneconomical to plan a protracted seduction with no guarantee of success when, for a smaller monetary outlay, he is assured of the product without delay.

2) Prostitution offers a convenient outlet for those wishing to avoid emotional attachment or the worry of possible pregnancy or other sequelae. 3) Call girls may be placed at the disposal of businessmen to influence favorably their business decisions, or at conventions. 4) Some married men may have strong sexual drives but encounter only limited response from their wives.

Function of Prostitution

In considering the function of prostitution it is relevant to consider three questions: why women become prostitutes, *i.e.,* what is the process of prostitution; the relationship of prostitution to other sexual outlets, *e.g.,* marriage; and why men visit prostitutes?

It has been suggested that women resort to prostitution because of hypersexuality. This theory is untenable, both on theoretical grounds and from observations of practicing prostitutes. Emotional involvement in sexual acts is a serious liability for the prostitute; it impairs her efficiency to process a large number of clients in a short time. The highly sexed woman may be promiscuous, but it is inappropriate for her to become a prostitute if she is more interested in sex than in money.

Despite this mercenary interest, it is equally misleading to consider that women always enter prostitution because of economic necessity. In some environments, increasing economic hardship influences a proportion of the population toward prostitution. In the same community, there will always be many women in even greater financial distress who resist prostituting themselves.[51] Sieff[52] supports this view: "Promiscuity, therefore, is not related to economics. A woman may sell herself for a drink or a meal, or a mink or a car."

While in nineteenth-century England married women were often forced to prostitute themselves to feed their families,[53] motivation from economic necessity in modern times is confined to periods of social upheaval usually associated with war. Under the harsh living conditions in Italy in World War II, women sold themselves and their daughters for paltry sums or a little food.[54] A large proportion of Russian refugees in China in the 1930s were forced into prostitution because they were barred from any other employment. Of 800 Russian prostitutes in Shanghai in 1937, only 5 percent had been prostitutes in Russia.[55] In Korea, over 99 percent of prostitutes had assumed their occupation only after becoming refugees.[56] The abolition of suttee in India produced many Hindu widows who were forced into prostitution to survive.[57]

The parttime clandestine prostitute may earn a relatively high salary in her respectable occupation. Likewise, "the wives of petty tradesmen and others similarly situated resorted to prostitution as an extra source of income rather than from necessity."[58] The prostitute has a desire for material possessions and luxurious living.[59] Workers on the Tyneside scheme[60] considered laziness was a marked characteristic of the prostitutes they encountered. They concluded that craving for luxury rather than economic need was their main motivation. Desire for excitement and luxuries have been noted by other authors.[61] Tait considered that love of dress, desire for property, and indolence were the major causes of prostitution.[62] The purpose of the prostitute's earnings is not to convert a life of hardship to one of comfort but rather to replace a comfortable life with a luxurious one.

Against this background, any effort to reduce the temptation of prostitution by making more employment available and raising salaries is inappropriate. No ordinary occupation, available to the average woman, can hope to compete with prostitution in terms of economic return for work performed. "Working six good days, I can make more than $1,000, tax free. It's the easiest way I know to make that kind of money."[63] As Davis[64] comments, in view of the high income for the relatively easy work, "the interesting question is not why so many women become prostitutes, but why so few of them do."

The answer is twofold: first, the payment is for loss of self-esteem or social standing. Secondly, for a large proportion of the population it is not easy to establish a successful prostitution business. Most societies condemn commercial prostitution on moral grounds. The prostitute faces loss of respect from her family, her peers, and the rest of society. Furthermore, this loss of respect is irreversible. Abandoning the profession after one or two years will not redeem the prostitute in the eyes of the community. The puritan might express this concept by saying she has sold her soul:

> All the organizations engaged in the reclamation of the prostitute report the same insuperable difficulties in obtaining society's acceptance of the reformed whore. . . . In Britain this was, and remains, one of the fundamental realities of the prostitute's life. The sin is irrevocable.[65]

Henriques makes the interesting comment that this rejection is almost entirely at the female level. A contemporary businessman's mistress will be accepted by his colleagues but not by their wives. In the past some prostitutes have overcome their beginnings (e.g., Nell Gwyn whose grandson became bishop, and Celeste Mogador who married a man subsequently the French Consul General in Melbourne), but such cases are remarkably rare.

Clinard[66] comments, "Most girls of this type have lived in local communities, such as slums, where sexual promiscuity has been approved or at least condoned. . . . The important other factor is association with persons on the fringe of prostitution." Bryan[67] reported that 96 percent of call girls had contact with prostitutes prior to entering their profession. A bad home situation where the mother may be poor and a prostitute is an important cause of prostitution.[68] Adler[69] mentions a mother and daughter working in the same brothel but gives no indication of the incidence of this phenomenon. (In nineteenth-century India, prostitution was largely hereditary.)[70] For girls without this type of background, becoming a successful prostitute may be quite difficult. In any case, it requires considerable effort. Certainly it cannot be equated with experimenting with alcohol, cigarettes, or drugs, nor does it compare with an array of other occupations in which a trial period is possible. In this respect, prostitution is by no means unique, but because of its clandestine nature, establishing an initial clientele is even more difficult for prostitutes.

The process of prostitution usually arises from a familiarity with others associated with the profession. Having gained acceptance to the profession, the prostitute must serve an apprenticeship to accumulate all facets of the *modus operandi* of the trade. The proficient prostitute must then acquire a clientele.

The concept that prostitutes once lured into the profession under false pretences are then unable to leave due to blackmail or physical coercion is hardly valid. It is true that many prostitutes find it difficult or impossible to leave their occupation. This may be related to debts to madams or other associates, but this bond has its origins in psychological factors rather than physical ones.

There is a popular concept that prostitution is necessary to cater to the sexual excesses of some men or the requirements of itinerants so that respectable women are not molested or wives not degraded. Hijmans[71] quotes many such views from diverse sources:

> Herself the supreme type of vice, she is ultimately the most efficient guardian of virtue. But for her, the unchallenged purity of countless homes would be polluted . . . ;
> I want to declare that, even in broad daylight, I would not dare to walk about with my wife and daughters in a city without brothels;
> Where six or seven thousand sailors arrive at once, as often happens at Amsterdam, that have seen none but their own sex for many months together, how is it to be supposed that honest women should walk the streets unmolested, if there were no Harlots to be had at reasonable prices. . . . It is manifest that there is a necessity of sacrificing one part

of woman-kind to preserve the other, and prevent a filthiness of a more heinous nature.

The function of the prostitute guarantees a certain social benefit as it diverts the sensuality of man from society and it prevents crime.

Hijmans himself summarizes, "Denunciation of the evil of prostitution and, in the same breath, affirmation of its indispensability has gone through the ages in Christian society."

While these views are debatable, it cannot be denied that both the sexual standards and the behavior of a society have a direct influence on prostitution. Marriage, prostitution, and promiscuity for pleasure are interrelated, and any change in one inevitably influences the others. Davis[72] describes how rigid standards may benefit prostitution: "By defining certain coital techniques as immoral and hence out of bounds for wives and sweethearts, the moral order gives an advantage to the prostitute." A relaxation of the moral code with a consequent rise in promiscuity for pleasure adversely affects not only marriage but also prostitution and weakens the motivation for marriage. The permissive society is the common enemy of both marriage and prostitution. The realization that prostitution may be reduced or even eliminated by increasing permissiveness provides the moralist with a dilemma. To him, the concept of sex purely for pleasure is as unacceptable as the commercial commodity it replaces.

Men go to prostitutes primarily because it is the most convenient method for a particular sexual outlet at a particular time. A consideration of the clients of prostitutes indicates the diversity of reasons for this convenience. There may be no other women available; simplicity and economy may be factors. Alternatively, the impersonal anonymous nature of sex with a prostitute may be the major attraction. This appeals to those who for real or imagined reasons have difficulty in establishing social relations with women. It appeals also to those wishing to indulge perverse cravings or abnormal ventures into eroticism which might offend close acquaintances.

For these reasons the demand for prostitution is broadly based and inextinguishable. That is why, when prostitution is outlawed, it falls into a category of crime that is notoriously hard to control—the type in which one of the guilty parties is the ordinary law-abiding citizen, who is receiving an illicit service.[73]

Prostitution and Venereal Disease

The role of prostitution in the dissemination of venereal disease has varied through the ages and varies from one country to another.

Table 5-1 demonstrates this relationship in some countries in recent times. The role of prostitution depends largely on the extent to which it provides for the promiscuous outlet and on the relative infectivity of the prostitutes. In general, prostitution is the major outlet in Eastern and developing countries, and the prostitutes there are heavily infested.[74] In Western countries, promiscuity for pleasure is becoming the major source of infection. Among merchant seamen, the pickup for no fee is the most common type of encounter in the United States and Europe. House prostitution is the most common in Mexico, Japan, West Indies, Central and South America, India, and Africa.[75] In one study among Liverpool men, only 13 percent had been infected by prostitutes as compared to 50 percent by "good-time girls' and 37 percent by acquaintances.[76] Prostitutes contribute little to the venereal disease problem in New Zealand.[77]

TABLE 5-1   PROSTITUTION AND VENEREAL DISEASE IN VARIOUS COUNTRIES[a]

Country	Year	Comment
Ceylon	1956	46.3% VD from prostitutes
Columbia	1956	83.4% from prostitutes
France	1965	30–40% of syphilis from prostitutes
Germany	1964	VD 50–100 times more frequent in prostitutes
Italy	1964	Prostitution most important source VD
Japan	1958	Prostitutes the source of 70% VD
Lebanon	1965	57% streetwalkers had VD
Portugal	1964	26.5% prostitutes had VD
		Prostitution important source VD
Thailand	1965	Prostitutes main source VD
United Kingdom	1959	2.6% prison prostitutes had VD
	1954	35.7% VD from prostitutes
United States	1967	10–15% syphilis patients named prostitutes as source
Holland	1967	42% VD from prostitutes
Western Pacific	1968	80–90% of VD from prostitutes

[a] Guthe T, Willcox RR: The international incidence of venereal disease, Int Health Conf Edinburgh, 21–25, 1970. Willcox RR: Factors leading to a failure of control of gonorrhea, Br J Prev Soc Med 16: 113, 1962. Willcox RR: Prostitution and venereal disease, Br J Vener Dis 38: 37, 1962

Conclusions

The layman when confronted with problems associated with prostitution may ask what should be done about prostitution. Some individuals might consider it more appropriate to ask if anything should be done about prostitution. It is clear that this must be answered in the affirmative. Providing we accept the desirability of at least some social regulations, almost any community occurrence, be it alcoholism, traffic accidents, or marriage, can profit from better understanding and appropriate action. Because of its diversity and its definite sociological role, it is inappropriate to consider prostitution as an evil, either necessary or unnecessary, against which we must defend society.

In addition to desirable innovations, it is equally important to consider the question, what should *not* be done about prostitution.

The prospect of eliminating prostitution. The only method by which prostitution can be eliminated is to eliminate the demand for it. This would involve a revolutionary and almost inconceivable change of social standards and behavior. Certainly it could not be achieved by statutory demands imposed on society. The so-called reduction, suppression, or elimination of prostitution that occurs in various societies from time to time is usually an indication that prostitution has either changed its form or given way to other sexual outlets which the moralist may find equally unacceptable.

The legality of prostitution. The more undesirable aspects of prostitution are associated with its encounters with the law. To make prostitution *per se* illegal is undesirable on two counts. First, it is unjust to the prostitute who is made the scapegoat for the phenomenon, whereas her client who is equally involved goes free. Secondly, it catalyzes the exploitation of prostitutes by madams, criminal syndicates, and the police. Much of the exploitation of the prostitute amounts to blackmail, which depends in turn on the illegality of the profession. Because of this, the prostitute is in no position to seek the aid of law-enforcing authorities while her occupation operates outside the guidelines imposed by the statutes under which these authorities operate.

To make prostitution legal does not mean that society must accept brothels, streetwalkers, or any other particular facet of the profession. The question of what forms prostitution should take is much more complex and must vary from one society to another.

There is general agreement that the law should curb those who exploit prostitutes or incorporate prostitution into criminal organization. In practice this may prove difficult, particularly when those involved in law enforcement tend to become involved in the corruption they are supposed to be eliminating. Making prostitution *per se* legal destroys probably the most potent tool the exploiters possess.

Prostitution and venereal disease. The contribution of prostitution to the venereal disease problem varies greatly from one society to another. As promiscuous sex for pleasure supplants prostitution, the latter makes a smaller contribution to the incidence of infection. It is promiscuity, whether commercial or for pleasure, that facilitates the spread of venereal disease.

Both the type of prostitution and the type of clients have a significant influence on venereal disease control. The prostitute who services the traveler has the greatest potential for harm. Infection may be disseminated widely throughout the country (or internationally), and the source is much more difficult to trace.

The routine enforced medical examination of the prostitute is a pointless exercise that does not contribute to infectious disease control. Where the venereal disease rate is high in a prostitute population, mass antibiotic treatment of the population is likely to be highly effective, although it can be opposed as an infringement of the rights of the individual. Acceptance of the prostitute as an individual and interest in her physical and psychological needs may be expected to induce greater cooperation from her profession. Certainly little impact on the venereal disease problem can be expected without this cooperation.

Chapter Six

Homosexuality and Homosexual Behavior

Definitions

Much of the confusion and disagreement on homosexuality, both in the literature and in the public mind, arises from the failure to distinguish between "homosexuality" and "homosexual behavior." The former involves sexual preference and conditions of arousal. The latter relates purely to objective phenomena without regard to motivation or psychological factors. Although many homosexuals are expected to indulge in homosexual behavior, these two components are discrete independent entities having vastly different sociological significance. Homosexuals may go through life without experiencing any overt homosexual behavior. Individuals indulging in frequent homosexual behavior may have no homosexual tendencies whatsoever. This fact is clearly illustrated by groups of male prostitutes who indulge in fellatio with homosexuals but will react against their clients with violence if there is any effort by the customer to diversify this behavior or respond to the prostitute with caresses or endearments during the contact.[1]

It has been suggested that individuals occupy a continuum from complete heterosexuality through bisexuality to complete homosexuality. Although this concept is undoubtedly valid, it does not clarify the distribution of individuals along this continuum and is of limited practical application. It is more practical to classify individuals as homosexual, heterosexual, or bisexual.

Homosexuals are individuals who are erotically aroused predominantly by members of their own sex and who have a marked preference for sexual experience with these members.

Heterosexuals are individuals whose erotic arousal and sexual preference focus on members of the opposite sex.

Bisexuals are individuals who can derive full erotic satisfaction with members of either sex and do not have a strong preference for the sex of the partner. Bisexuality must be excessively rare, although, of course, bisexual behavior is very common. It may be considered adaptively more stable than either exclusive heterosexual or homosexual behavior.

Many other terms used to describe sexuality are either redundant or contradictory. They tend to be confusing rather than clarifying. Exclusive or obligatory homosexuals are simply homosexuals. Overt homosexuals are homosexuals who indulge in homosexual behavior; covert homosexuals do not. *Facultative homosexuality* is a contradiction of terms since facultative homosexual behavior is the phenomenon usually considered, *viz.,* sexual experience between members of the same sex when persons of the opposite sex are not available. These individuals are not homosexual, of course, for their preference is for heterosexual behavior. The term *latent homosexuality* introduces nebulous psychological and philosophic concepts into a classification already overloaded with philosophy at the expense of science.

The terms *active* and *passive homosexuality* are particularly misleading because they tend to perpetuate the myth that homosexuals fall into two distinct categories—those filling the male role and those filling the female role. In actual practice no such distinction exists. Most homosexuals tend to indulge in an array of sexual behaviors of both active and passive nature. It is true that some homosexuals do have a preference for certain types of behavior but then so do many heterosexuals. It serves little purpose to attach false significance to such preference. The concept of male/female roles in homosexuality is a myth of analysis by heterosexuals. Many homosexual men will verify that they are not attracted to effeminate men. The reason is that they want a man and not a woman. In a hostile community, there are other reasons why homosexuals are reluctant to associate with those who are indiscreet in their behavior.

In contrast, there are many settings where role-playing in homosexual behavior is carried to extremes. From time to time various primitive societies have coped with a scarcity of females by forcing males to play the role of housewife in every detail. Castration has sometimes been used as an aid to feminize the partner who will be utilized in an exclusively passive role. These phenomena really belong to the area of facultative homosexual behavior rather than homosexuality, since this conduct is motivated by the desire for a substitute female rather than by preference for a male partner. It might be argued in fact that the establishment of male and female roles with pronounced efforts to masculinize and feminize the respective partners is incompatible with true homosexuality.

Homosexuality

Prevalence

Accurate statistics on the incidence of homosexuality are not available. Homosexual behavior, both throughout the animal kingdom and among human societies, is very common. To relate this behavior to homosexuality, as some authors customarily do, grossly and erroneously inflates the extent of homosexuality. Ford and Beach[2] found that 64 percent of the primitive societies they studied accepted some form of homosexual activity as normal. The literature abounds with accounts of homosexual behavior in societies throughout history. Homosexual experiences in adolescence are commonplace. Kinsey[3] found that 37 percent of males had some overt homosexual behavior in their adult life; 13 percent had more homosexual than heterosexual behavior for at least three years; and 4 percent had exclusively homosexual experiences. This information tells us little about the prevalence of homosexuality but, until more precise knowledge is available, it seems reasonable to assume that approximately 5 percent of males in Western society are homosexuals.

Etiology

The diversity of theories relating to the etiology of homosexuality testifies to our state of ignorance on this subject. No theory is applicable to all homosexuals.

Clinically, however, one is impressed by the number of homosexuals who have had disturbed parental relationships in their formative years. This is one facet upon which there is reasonably consistent agreement in the literature. Frequently a weak or absent father coupled with a dominant, possessive mother produces a poor paternal image for identification, while bringing about an intimate mother-son relationship. It has been postulated that intense feelings of conflict arising from this relationship produce a neurotic fear of heterosexuality. Sexual desires are thus directed toward members of the same sex.

This situation rarely arises from default or simple ignorance on the part of the parents but is a result of definite pathologic relationships. Bieber has clearly summarized this situation:

> In the majority of instances the father was explicitly detached or hostile. In only a minority of cases was paternal destructiveness affected through indifference or default. A fatherless child is deprived of the important paternal contribution to normal development; however, only few homosexuals in our sample had been fatherless children. Relative absence of the father, necessitated by occupational demands or unusual exigencies, is not in itself pathogenic. A good father-son relationship and a mother who is an affectionate, admiring wife provide the son with the basis for a positive image of the father during periods of separation. We have come to the conclusion that a constructive, supportive, warmly related father precludes the possibility of a homosexual son; he acts as a neutralizing, protective agent should the mother make seductive or closebinding attempts.[4]

The Psychiatric Status of Homosexuality

It is of considerable importance to assess whether or not homosexuality is pathologic. There is no doubt that the majority of the populace in Western society consider the abnormality of this phenomenon as beyond question. This view is of little relevance, however, since these same people consider homosexual behavior as being equally pathologic. Because of the widespread occurrence of such behavior in the animal kingdom, throughout various societies, and in the normal development of healthy individuals, this judgment is not scientifically valid. Western society's approach to sexual matters is so conservative and steeped in emotion and ignorance that its judgments are often merely an indictment of its own prejudice and intolerance.

It has been argued that homosexuality is "unnatural" because it is contrary to the primary function of sex—reproduction of the species. It could be countered, of course, that, where overpopulation is a threat, homosexuality acts as an adaptive process to reduce the proportion of the population contributing to reproduction. In ancient Greece, for example, homosexual behavior and the exposure of infants can both be regarded as responses to overpopulation.

More valid criticism of homosexuality has been made on the grounds of the nature of homosexuals themselves. It is misleading to consider that the only difference between homosexuals and heterosexuals is their sexual preference. The homosexual is very often a lonely individual who seems almost incapable of forming long-term intimate relationships. He also seems to have trouble in maintaining harmonious relationships with women in day-to-day living. The promiscuity of the homosexual is even more significant in a hostile community. The quest for new partners which this preference necessitates is hazardous and has a considerable bearing on the social organization of homosexuals. The generally unhappy life of the homosexual has led many people, including some homosexuals, to conclude that no one would choose to be a homosexual; all would change to heterosexuality if they could. This is a fair statement for some homosexuals.

Proponents of homosexuality have countered that the maladjustment typical of homosexuality is due to harsh laws and an intolerant society. Most current laws on homosexuality are indefensible and are more in keeping with medieval ignorance than the sociological understanding one would expect in the twentieth century. While the normality of homosexuality is debatable, the pathologic nature of the behavior of some police officers who act as decoys to entrap homosexuals or go out of their way to persecute them is more certain. Unfortunately, there are other members of the community who also carry this type of intolerance to extremes. Against this background of societal prejudice, statutory law is much less important than many would consider it. Changes in the laws would protect homosexuals from legal sanctions (a significant improvement, of course), but so long as the social stigma remains, blackmail and other unpleasant concomitants will still exist.

The prevalence of homosexuality is considered by some as further support of the normality of homosexuality. This view is quoted by West,[5] "homosexuals are so numerous they cannot all be serious misfits or outstandingly peculiar." In fact, the prevalence of homosexuality has been inflated by the inclusion of normal homosexual behavior in considerations of this phenomenon. Prevalence in any case is not a valid criterion of normality. For instance, it cannot be argued that diseases are not pathologic merely because they are endemic. At a psychological level, racism or genocide are not necessarily normal or desirable merely because they are widely practiced and accepted in a particular society.

Many homosexuals are maladjusted, not because of their homosexual behavior, but because of their inability to experience satisfying heterosexual relationships. For some homosexuals at least, this inability has its origins in neurotic conflicts. Homosexuality is therefore merely an indicator of defective development of certain interpersonal relationships during maturation.

The ultimate and irrefutable plea for the normality of homosexuality is that all descriptions of homosexuals are based on a biased sample. Whether one studies homosexuals in prison, those encountered in medical practice, or persons from certain homophile organizations, it is unlikely that those encountered are representative of the total homosexual population. In fact, there is most likely a strong bias to the most maladjusted end of the spectrum. It may be argued that there are many homosexuals living quite contentedly; the fact that society is unaware of their existence is a mark of their adjustment in a hostile community. The presumptive existence of these individuals does not negate the observations about other homosexuals, however. For a truly balanced appraisal of homosexuality one would need a comparison of homosexuals and heterosexuals taken in random samples from a community where both have equal acceptance and are subjected to the same societal pressures. It is unlikely that the possibility for such a study will exist in the near future.

Management

There is no reason *per se* to attempt to convert homosexuals to heterosexuals. Certainly the likelihood of achieving this conversion except when the attempt is initiated by the patient is negligible. With respect to individual therapy, the approach to the homosexual does not differ from that to the heterosexual. If the patient is neurotic or maladjusted, he is given support to cope with these problems. His sexuality is viewed merely as a component that contributes to his problems.

In terms of social medicine, it is obvious that adverse laws and public prejudice make a significant contribution to the problems of the homosexual. It is this public prejudice which makes homosexuality, as distinct from homosexual behavior, a special problem in venereology. The stigma attached to homosexuality creates reluctance to report venereal infection or to volunteer the names of contacts for tracing purposes. Despite this reluctance, the clinician must make every effort to obtain the full cooperation of the patient in order that all contacts can be traced. In particular, one must be aware that there are often heterosexual as well as homosexual contacts for the one individual. Even when some homosexual contacts have been volunteered, the patient may still withhold the names of his more intimate associates.

Homosexual Behavior

Many homosexuals attempt to abstain from sexual relations and obtain sexual satisfaction from homosexual fantasy during masturbation. It is unwise to assign sexual orientation on this criterion alone. It is more appropriate to consider the total psychosexual adjustment of the individual.

Both homosexuals and nonhomosexuals may engage in overt homosexual behavior, but the significance of the behavior for venereology is quite different for the two groups. On the one hand, the homosexual, possibly because of his weaknesses in cementing stable interpersonal relationships, may be habitually promiscuous. In one study, only 6 percent of homosexuals had had fewer than 15 partners. Most relationships were "one night stands."[6] This behavior is conducive to the rapid, widespread dissemination of venereal disease. The difficulties of identifying contacts reduce the impact of control policies. The nonhomosexual, on the other hand, has both fewer partners and fewer sexual experiences. He is usually more reticent about his behavior, however, and may relate his infection to heterosexual behavior. If he is asymptomatic, he is reluctant to attend a clinic for precautionary rectal examination.

The sexual behavior pattern of homosexuals tends to vary with age and experience. The encounters of young inexperienced individuals usually involve mutual masturbation. Fellatio may also be practiced and some anal intercourse may be introduced. With increasing experience there is less need to resort to masturbation and more sophisticated techniques predominate. Probably the majority of those using anal intercourse have some experience of both the active and passive roles.

An increase in homosexual behavior can be anticipated if partners of the opposite sex are not readily available: at sea, in prison, and in many developing countries where large indigenous work forces are transported from rural areas to meet the factory or domestic demands of rapid urban expansion. Armed forces are traditionally intolerant of homosexual behavior and exclude or persecute its practitioners.[7] In the nineteenth-century British navy the penalty was death.[8] In practice, homosexuals are excluded from most modern armies. Most soldiers have an aggressive outspoken antagonism to homosexuals or homosexuality. Exposure of a homosexual results in such widespread ridicule that his life becomes unbearable. In confined camp areas, with their lack of privacy, the risk of disclosure of any homosexual approach or union is too great for most homosexually inclined individuals to accept. For this reason homosexual behavior rarely features significantly in studies on military personnel.[9]

The increasing implication of homosexual behavior in the transmission of venereal disease is probably related to increasing honesty and frankness rather than to increased incidence of this behavior. Although many cases of gonorrhea result from homosexual contact, these form a relatively small proportion of the total incidence of the disease. In many areas, however, the majority of syphilitic infections are transmitted by homosexual behavior.[10] A large proportion of Donovanosis infections is also related to homosexual behavior.

A marked reduction in homosexually transmitted infection must occur if venereal disease is to be controlled. This reduction will be achieved only if homosexuals have a greater understanding of their susceptibility to venereal infection and cooperate in achieving control. The venereologist's role is to provide homosexuals with this knowledge of venereal infection and to create a favorable clinic environment that will induce cooperation.

Chapter Seven

The
Venereal
Diseases

Introduction

A number of texts cover the clinical aspects of the venereal diseases comprehensively.[1-3] This chapter briefly summarizes the salient features of these illnesses.

Table 7-1 shows the incidence of sexually transmitted diseases seen in hospital venereal disease clinics in England,[4] and it illustrates some features of the disease spectrum encountered there. These conditions may be grouped into various categories.

Functional Conditions

Many patients seen in clinics do not have sexually transmitted infection. Up to 50 percent may have no evidence of any infection. Some of these patients present as a result of contact tracing. Others come in for a routine check after intercourse. Still others will show marked anxiety or neurotic manifestations related to their possible exposure to venereal infection. In extreme cases the patient may be so obsessed with the idea that he has acquired venereal infection or that previous infection has not been cured that he resists reassurance to the contrary. For a variety of complex reasons, men contribute disproportionately to those without VD who attend venereal disease clinics.[5]

TABLE 7-1 SEXUALLY TRANSMITTED DISEASE: NEW CASES PER
100,000 POPULATION SEEN AT HOSPITAL CLINICS IN ENGLAND IN 1972

	Male	Female
Candidiasis	19.34	107.16
Nonspecific infection	277.65	60.61
Viral		
Herpes simplex	13.84	5.31
Condylomata acuminata	45.54	23.42
Molluscum contagiosum	2.03	0.74
Bacterial		
Gonorrhea	155.64	77.10
Chancroid	0.21	0.01
Donovanosis	0.01	0.01
LGV	0.24	0.02
Spirochetal		
Early syphilis	6.00	1.25
Protozoal		
Trichomoniasis	6.82	73.38
Metazoal		
Scabies	9.93	2.25
Pediculosis	13.45	4.50
Other Conditions		
Requiring treatment	101.85	39.32
Not requiring treatment	208.90	110.19

Urethritis

Urethritis is the most common venereal infection of males. It is frequently distributed fairly evenly between infections of gonococcal and nongonococcal etiology.

Penile Ulceration

The relative incidence of various forms of penile ulceration varies greatly according to geographical location and clinic population. The most common cause of penile ulceration is simple trauma. Probably only a few of those patients with traumatic ulcers attend a venereal disease clinic. They may use home remedies or consult their own doctors. In populations with greater concern about venereal diseases, a higher proportion of patients with traumatic lesions will attend a clinic. Of course, a traumatic ulcer may be superinfected with a specific sexually transmitted organism. Chancroid, Donovanosis, and LGV are common in some tropical and subtropical countries, but they are rare in most Western countries including the United States. The prevalence of syphilis varies greatly from one clinic to another, but is rarely responsible for more than a small proportion of penile ulcers.

Herpes genitalis is probably the most common specific cause of penile ulceration, but a conclusive diagnosis is often not possible in many clinical settings. Balanitis may vary in severity from mild erythema of the glans to widespread confluent ulceration of the glans and adjacent penis. Although *Candida* and a variety of bacteria can be isolated from these lesions, the primary etiology usually relates to the physical condition (moisture and cleanliness) of the glans. The incidence depends largely on the type of population considered.

Venereal Disease in Women

Because of differences in both anatomy and pathology, fewer women seek treatment for venereal infections in clinics. Most women with these infections attend clinics because of contact tracing efforts by their infected sex partner or clinic staff. Of those patients who attend because of vaginal discharge, a substantial proportion have trichomoniasis, candidiasis, and nonspecific cervicitis. Finally, nongonococcal urethritis, which is the most common venereal disease in men, is not a distinct clinical entity in women.

Miscellaneous Conditions

An array of other diseases will usually be encountered. Some of these may be acquired by sexual intercourse, some are related to any form of body contact, and others are purely dermatologic conditions unrelated in any way to sexual behavior. Some patients are greatly concerned about the infectivity of genital lesions, but it is not possible to provide precise estimates for some conditions.

The common conditions encountered include condyloma acuminatum, molluscum contagiosum, scabies, pediculosis pubis, and fungal infections. Phimosis, paraphimosis and a range of congenital anomalies are also commonly encountered.

General Features of the Venereal Diseases

Some features of epidemiology or management are shared by many or all of the venereal diseases.

Age Distribution

Most venereal infections occur predominantly in the 15–30 age group. There is an increasing awareness of infection in even younger groups. Infection in children under one year often occurs from non-sexual contact, but most infections past this age are acquired sexually.

Sex Distribution

For many of these diseases, the reported male cases exceed the reported female cases. This may be partly an artificial result stemming from diminished case findings for various reasons. A decreasing male: female sex ratio is sometimes suggested as an indicator of improved contact tracing. In some communities, however, a limited number of women may provide sexual outlet for a larger number of men. Infections transmitted by homosexual contact may contribute to an excess of male infections. In many environments, for instance, 50 percent or more of reported syphilis infections occur in homosexuals.

Sites of Infection

Most infections involve the genitalia, but infections of the rectum and pharynx are also common. Primary infection of other anatomic sites is rare, but with several diseases, systemic dissemination from the primary site may produce lesions throughout the body.

Complication of Pregnancy

The potential sequelae of several of these diseases (*e.g.*, syphilis, gonorrhea, herpes, CMV infection) are magnified when the pregnant woman is infected.[6]

Coexistence of Several Sexually Transmitted Diseases

Individuals with one venereal infection are usually in a high-risk group for the other diseases prevalent in the same environment. Consequently, multiple screening should be employed in VD clinics.

Evaluation of Sex Partners

The sex partners of patients with any venereal infection should be medically evaluated. This is essential not only to prevent further dissemination throughout the community, but also to minimize the chances of reinfection for the original patient.

Gonococcal Infection

History

Gonorrhea has its origins in antiquity, being known to the early Chinese (in the time of Emperor Huang-ti, 2637 B.C.). There are many references in the Bible almost certainly alluding to this illness, *e.g.*,

Leviticus 15:1, "A running issue out of his flesh." Although the disease was known to Hippocrates in 400 B.C., Galen in 130 A.D. was responsible for the name gonorrhea, meaning "flow of seed," for the condition was thought to be a flow of semen unrelated to intercourse.

The *Diplococcus* was first identified and named the gonococcus by Neisser in 1879. It was first grown on artificial media by Bumm in 1885. The use of selective culture medium was described by Thayer and Martin in 1964.

Pathology

Neisseria gonorrhoeae are spherical or ovoid Gram-negative organisms, with a diameter of 0.6–1.0 μ. These usually appear as intracellular diplococci in smears prepared directly from infected sites. Best cultured on media that have been enriched with whole blood, hemoglobin, ascitic fluid, or serum, they grow most readily at 35–36°C in a moist atmosphere containing 3 percent–20 percent carbon dioxide. Gonococci are not motile, flagellated, or hemolytic. Typically they form 1–2mm round, greyish, glistening, oxidase-positive colonies after 24–48 hours growth. The organism will ferment glucose but not fructose, maltose, sucrose, or mannitol, a characteristic which differentiates it from all other *Neisseria*.

When grown on solid media, *N. gonorrhoeae* produces at least four morphologically distinct types of colonies. Types I and II are virulent for man, are more resistant to phagocytosis than are types III and IV, and are covered by hairlike surface projections called pili, which are absent from the avirulent types. The gonococcus possesses an endotoxin, similar to that of the meningococcus, which may contribute to pathogenicity.

The gonococcus has a predilection for columnar epithelium, but transitional and squamous epithelium are sometimes affected. The anatomic sites commonly infected by direct inoculation include the urethra, anal canal, conjunctivae, pharynx, and endocervix. Local spread from the primary focus may produce bartholinitis, pelvic inflammatory disease (PID), and perihepatitis in the female, and paraurethral abscess, prostatitis, and epididymitis in the male. Dissemination by gonococcemia may occur. Subsequent localization of infection may produce arthritis, dermatitis, endocarditis, meningitis, and hepatitis.

Clinical Features

Male urethritis. The incubation period is commonly 4 or 5 days and, in over 80 percent of cases, symptoms develop within 8 days of sexual contact.[8] The asymptomatic infective state may last for weeks or months, however. Probably 1 percent–3 percent of infected men remain asymptomatic. The classic features of infection are reddening and edema of the urethral meatus, followed within 12 hours by dysuria and urethral discharge, initially mucoid or mucopurulent, but rapidly becoming thick, creamy, and profuse. Any or all of these features may be modified or absent, and gonococcal urethritis can only be excluded by a urethral culture.

Urethritis may resolve spontaneously. The average duration of the untreated infection is 8 weeks. Ninety-five percent will become asymptomatic within 6 months. Gonococcal prostatitis (characterized by pelvic pain, fever, and occasionally urinary retention or hematuria) and epididymitis (usually unilateral and characterized by pain, swelling, and tenderness) used to occur in about 15 percent of untreated infections. In the antibiotic era, these afflict less than 3 percent of infected men.

Gonorrhea is the cause of a variable proportion of urethritis as it is encountered in different environments. It may account for as little as 10 percent of the urethritis seen among white college students,[9] to as much as 60 percent of that seen in black men attending a VD clinic.[10] While nongonococcal urethritis tends to have an incubation period of 2–3 weeks and is usually associated with less florid symptoms, the two conditions may be clinically indistinguishable.

Endocervicitis. Gonococcal endocervicitis probably produces symptoms in less than 50 percent of infected women. Some infected women, however, will have a coincidental vaginal discharge from candidiasis, trichomoniasis, or nonspecific cervicitis. Gonococcal infection may produce increased vaginal discharge, often purulent, or dysuria, frequency, labial tenderness, and dyspareunia. Examination often reveals thick, purulent discharge issuing from the cervical canal. Although not diagnostic, a history of purulent discharge and dysuria 5–10 days following intercourse suggests gonococcal infection. Bartholinitis in the sexually active age group should be considered gonococcal until proven otherwise.

Pelvic inflammatory disease (PID). Proximal spread from the endocervix to the endometrium, fallopian tubes, ovarian surface, and pelvic peritoneum is the most serious local complication of gonococcal infection. It probably affects about 15 percent of the infected women. Dull, aching, or occasionally cramping lower abdominal pain, sometimes beginning or exacerbated at menstruation, occurs in over 90 percent of affected women. A mild increase in vaginal discharge occurs in over 50 percent, menstrual irregularities in one-third, and dysuria in about 10 percent of those affected. Examination may reveal adnexal tender-

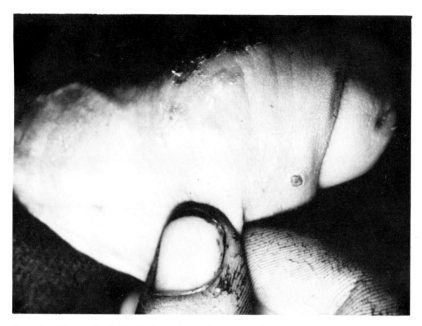

Plate 1. Herpes Genitalis. Early vesicular lesions on the penis. (Reproduced with permission from Technical Information Services, Center for Disease Control, Public Health Service, Dept. HEW).

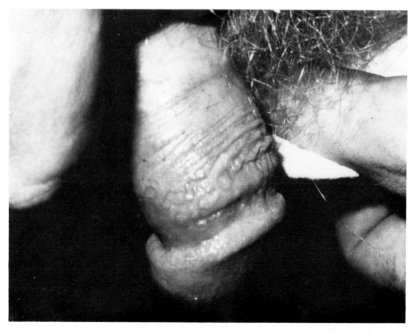

Plate 2. Herpes Genitalis. Multiple, shallow, uniformly sized subpreputial herpetic ulcers.

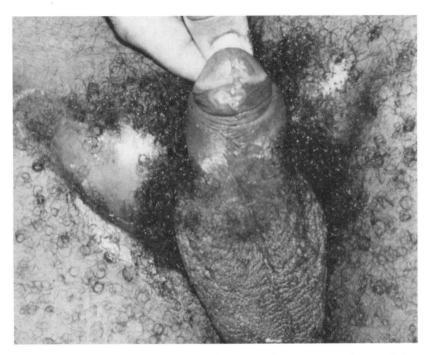

Plate 3. Donovanosis. Beefy frenular granuloma and subcutaneous granulomata of the penile shaft and inguinal regions.

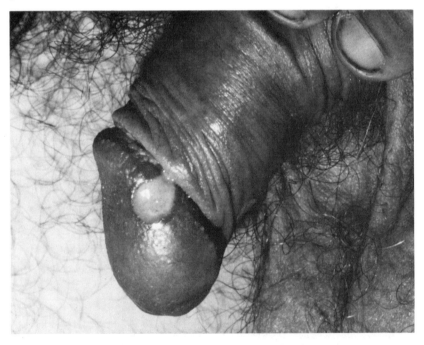

Plate 4. Chancroid. Erosive chancroidal ulcer of 3 days duration.

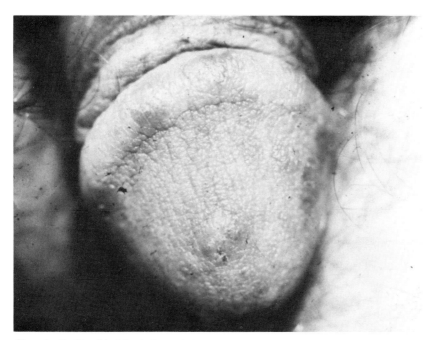

Plate 5. Scabies. Nodular lesions of the glans.

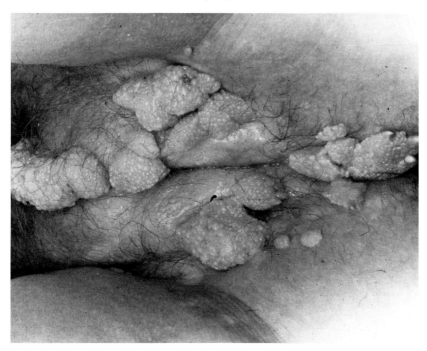

Plate 6. Condylomata acuminata. Fleshy filiform lesions of the vulva (Reproduced with permission from Technical Information Services, Center for Disease Control, Public Health Service, Dept. HEW).

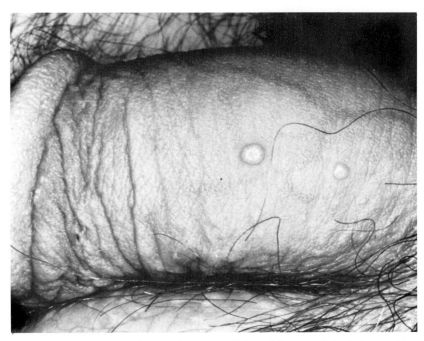

Plate 7. Molluscum contagiosum. The characteristic umbilication of the lesions enables clinical diagnosis. (Reproduced with permission of Medcom Inc., 2 Hammarskjold Plaza, New York, NY 10017).

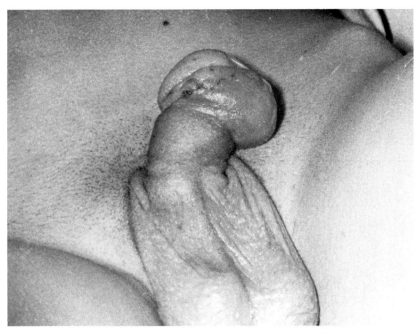

Plate 8. Severe preputial edema following fellatio. Teeth marks proximal to the coronal sulcus are visible.

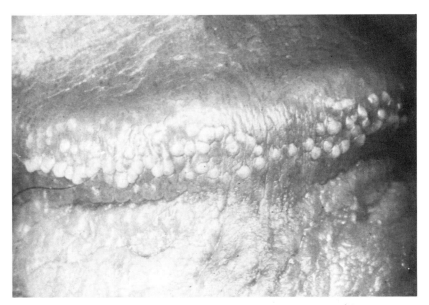

Plate 9. Pearly penile papules (Acral Angiofibromata). These white papules, commonly occurring in 1 to 3 rows around the coronal margin, are of no functional or pathological significance. They should not be confused with venereal condylomata. (Reproduced with permission from Medcom Inc., 2 Hammarskjold Plaza, New York, NY 10017)

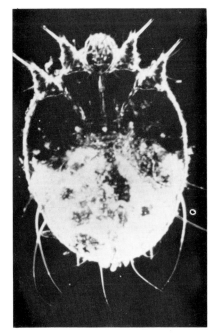

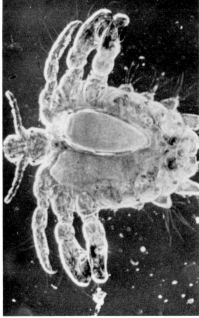

Plate 10. Sarcoptes scabiei (scabies mite). (Reproduced with permission from Reed and Carnrick, Kenilworth, New Jersey 07033)

Plate 11. Phthirus pubis (female)—the cause of pediculosis pubis. (Reproduced with permission from Reed and Carnrick, Kenilworth, New Jersey 07033)

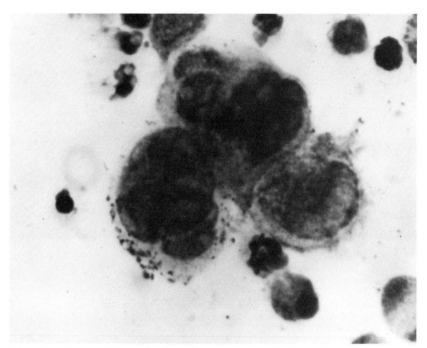

Plate 12. Characteristic multinucleate giant cells appearing in a Giemsa-stained smear prepared by scraping the base of a freshly ruptured vesicle of herpes genitalis.

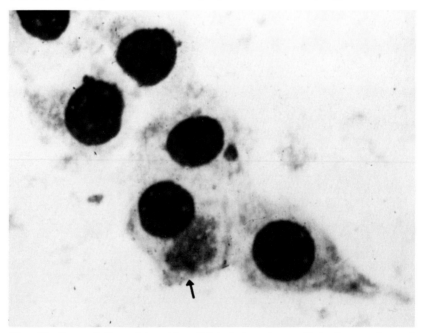

Plate 13. Brown iodine-staining chlamydial inclusions (arrowed) in the cytoplasm of tissue culture cells.

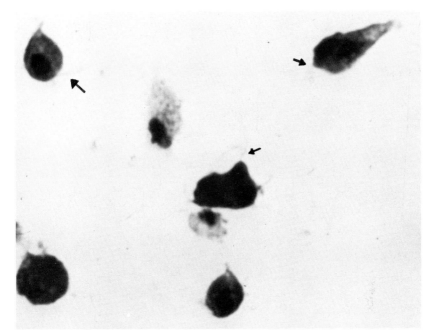

Plate 14. Trichomonads in a Giemsa-stained smear. The red-staining flagellae (arrowed) are readily seen opposite the pointed axostyle.

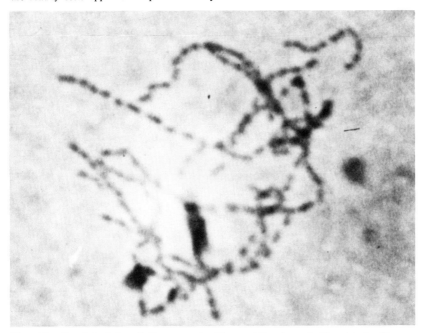

Plate 15. Tangled chains of Gram-negative Haemophilus ducreyi. (Reprinted with permission of Technical Information Services, Center for Disease Control, Public Health Service, Dept. HEW).

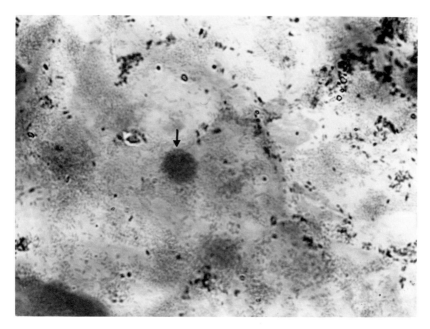

Plate 16. A typical vaginal smear of *Corynebacterium Vaginale* demonstrating the multitude of small Gram-negative bacilli granular clue cell (arrowed) scattered dark Gram-positive lactobacilli and absence of polymorphs.

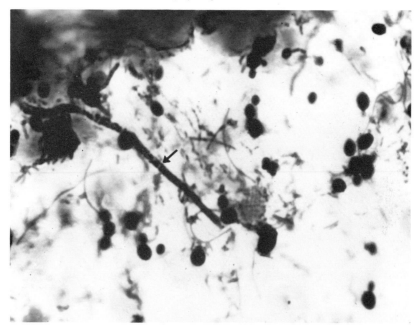

Plate 17. Gram stained vaginal smear demonstrating dense Gram-positive spores of *Candida Albicans*. The speckled hypha (arrowed) suggests a pathogenic role of the yeast.

ness, a palpable adnexal mass, and fever. Pain on movement of the cervix is common.

Pelvic inflammatory disease frequently recurs, and the probability of sterility or ectopic pregnancy increases with each recurrence. Even a single episode of PID impairs fertility in about 15 percent of the affected patients.

The precise role of the gonococcus in PID is not well understood. Although gonococci taken from the cervix may be cultured in up to 80 percent of patients presenting with an initial episode of PID, the culture positivity rate drops to 50 percent or less in patients who have had three or more recurrences. It is possible that other organisms such as anaerobes and other vaginal flora produce recurrent infection after gonococci have damaged the normal tubal epithelium.

Pelvic inflammatory disease may be an early complication of gonorrhea. In one series, 16 percent of the women with an uncomplicated infection developed PID at the time of their first period after acquiring the infection.

Gonococcal perihepatitis (Fitz-Hugh and Curtis syndrome). Gonococcal perihepatitis is virtually confined to women and probably occurs by direct extension from a pelvic focus. This syndrome consists of right upper quadrant pain, often referred to the right shoulder, hepatic tenderness, and transient elevation of liver enzymes. A friction rub in the right upper quadrant may accompany respiration. The oral cholecystogram may be transiently abnormal, making differentiation from acute cholecystitis difficult.

Anorectal infection. Rectal gonorrhea can produce a flagrant proctitis with a copious rectal discharge, tenesmus, and bloody diarrhea containing mucus and pus. Asymptomatic infection is more common. In mild symptomatic cases, slight rectal burning or pruritis may be the only complaint. These mild symptoms, however, are also common in those practicing anal intercourse who do not have gonococcal infection. The proctoscopic picture varies from flagrant cases resembling ulcerative colitis to essentially normal findings.

Pharyngeal infection. Pharyngeal infection may occasionally present as an exudative pharyngitis, but is usually asymptomatic. It is no more common among venereal disease clinic patients complaining of a sore throat than in those who do not.

Gonococcal conjunctivitis. Ophthalmia neonatorum classically appears as an intense redness and swelling of the conjunctivae and profuse purulent discharge within 3 days of birth, although application of local prophylactics may prolong the incubation period to over a week. It is bilateral in the majority of cases. If untreated, gross epithelial destruction may occur within 48 hours, and corneal ulceration may progress to panophthalmia or orbital cellulitis.

In the adult, an acute purulent conjunctivitis, unilateral in about two-thirds of cases, develops after an incubation period of about 3 days.

Disseminated gonococcal infection (DGI). Systemic dissemination occurs in 1 percent–3 percent of patients with gonorrhea. It occurs about twice as frequently in women as in men and is most frequently observed during pregnancy or at the time of menstruation. The disease often follows an asymptomatic genital infection or pharyngeal infection. It has been observed after an apparent isolated infection of the rectum.

This infection has two stages. Initially, there is frank gonococcal bacteremia. Blood cultures are positive in about 50 percent of the cases. In this stage, the patient is often febrile and may experience rigors. Skin lesions characteristic of septic vasculitis appear, usually on the extremities. They often involve the palms and soles. The lesions begin as papule but later become petechial. They may involute or may progress with the development of central vesicles, which soon become pustular and necrotic; gonococci may be demonstrated in their centers. The classic, fully developed lesion is usually located distally on an extremity. It consists of an erythematous or hemorrhagic area with a grey necrotic center. There are often only about six to ten lesions if the patients consult a physician soon after onset, but patients with 50 or more early lesions are occasionally seen.

While these skin lesions are developing, the patient almost always complains of polyarthralgia and may present with frank polyarthritis. The knees, wrists, hands, and elbows are most frequently involved; the joints usually lack sufficient effusion to permit successful aspiration. Tenosynovitis is characteristic; it may be detected by palpating the tendons at a slight distance from the joint or by having the patient move the tendons crossing an involved joint while the joint itself is immobilized by the examiner.

If the disease remains untreated, the patient may enter the second, or septic joint stage. Bacteremia ceases; blood cultures are usually negative; no new skin lesions develop. The polyarthritis disappears, and the infection tends to localize in a single joint. The affected joint develops a purulent effusion from which gonococci can usually be isolated. Accompanying tenosynovitis suggests a gonococcal etiology.

Meningitis and endocarditis each occur in about 2 percent–4 percent of cases of DGI. Gonococci have been identified in the spinal fluid from patients initially thought to have meningococcal infection.

Diagnosis

While the clinical presentation may strongly suggest gonorrhea in some cases of urethritis in men, gonococcal infection cannot be confidently diagnosed clinically in women. It can never be excluded in either sex without confirmatory laboratory aids.

The Gram stain is the preferred method for evaluating smears. This technique is highly specific and sensitive for gonorrhea in symptomatic men. It is reasonably specific, but lacks sensitivity in asymptomatic urethral infection, endocervical, or rectal infection. It is of no use in detecting pharyngeal infection.

The current culture medium of choice is a modification of the original Thayer–Martin formula, which contains vancomycin, colistin, and nystatin to prevent the growth of unwanted commensals, and trimethoprim to suppress the swarming of proteus, which is of particular importance in specimens taken from the rectum. Selective media will generally inhibit growth of nonpathogenic *Neisseria* but will permit the multiplication of *N. meningitidis* and some strains of *Moraxella.*

A carbon dioxide-enriched aerobic environment may be obtained by using a candle jar or by use of special flat culture plates containing a carbon dioxide-generating tablet which after inoculation are sealed in individual plastic bags.

Use of selective media and identification by typical colonial morphology, the oxidase reaction (production of a purple color when exposed to dimethyl or tetramethyl-p-phenylenediamine hydrochloride), and microscopic examination are over 99.5 percent specific for identifying gonococcal infection of the urethra, endocervix, or rectum. The sensitivity of endocervical culture is uncertain, but it is probably from 70 percent–90 percent.

Cultures taken from the pharynx or conjunctivae require further confirmation by sugar fermentation or by the fluorescent antibody staining of smears. Serologic diagnosis of gonorrhea is imperfectly developed.

Samples for cultures preferably should be plated directly, for the use of transport media decreases the yield obtained. For instance, with Stuart's medium, 5 percent of the samples are lost after 12 hours and 17 percent after 24 hours.[11] Attention to detail in collecting specimens is essential if optimum yields are to be obtained.

With symptomatic urethritis, fresh discharge may be collected on a platinum loop or cotton swab. In asymptomatic men, a saline-moistened calcium alginate swab or small cotton swab is inserted 4–5 cm into the anterior urethra. For endocervical samples, a cotton swab is inserted

1 cm into the cervical canal and gently rotated before removal. For rectal samples, the saline-moistened swab is inserted 2 cm into the anal canal and rotated against the anorectal mucosa. Pharyngeal samples are obtained by thorough swabbing of both tonsils or tonsillar fossae.

In men with symptomatic urethritis, the Gram smear is over 95 percent sensitive and specific.[12] Treatment should be initiated on the basis of this test—for gonorrhea if positive, for nongonococcal urethritis if negative. As the smear is at most only 70 percent sensitive, even when modified to give maximum sensitivity, in asymptomatic men,[13] a culture should always be performed. A positive smear, however, is an indication for immediate treatment for gonorrhea.

The Gram stain has a sensitivity of approximately 50 percent for gonococcal cervicitis and is highly specific only in experienced hands. Consequently, a culture is mandatory for the diagnosis of gonorrhea in the female. In most cases, treatment should be given before the results of culture are known. Immediate treatment should be given to those who have a positive endocervical Gram stain, those who are contacts of known cases, or those in whom gonorrhea is suspected on epidemiologic grounds.

Although the Gram stain is of some value, rectal gonorrhea should be diagnosed only on the basis of culture results. Antibiotic therapy should be given immediately if the smear is positive. Culture alone is inadequate for diagnosing pharyngeal infection, as only a minority of *Neisseria* grown on Thayer–Martin medium from this site are gonococci. The specific techniques of sugar fermentation or fluorescent antibody staining must be used as confirmatory procedures.

Gram stains, culture, and specific techniques should be used for examining conjunctival discharge. Although the diagnosis is confirmed only by specific techniques, again, immediate treatment should be initiated on the basis of a positive smear or culture.

Fluorescent antibody staining is the most sensitive method of detecting gonococci in vesicular or pustular skin lesions. It detects 60 percent of the cases, compared with 15 percent by either Gram stain or culture. Culture of joint fluid is positive in up to 75 percent of patients in the septic-joint stage, but in less than 10 percent of patients in the bacteremic phase. When DGI is suspected, attempted isolation of gonococci from the genitalia, pharynx, and rectum is essential. Isolation of gonococci from any of these sites, in the presence of the typical clinical syndrome of DGI, constitutes acceptable criteria for diagnosis.

Cultures should always be used to test the cure at any site, but a positive smear is an indication for immediate retreatment.

Treatment

Because of changing sensitivity in the gonococcus and because of the introduction of new antibiotics, the recommended therapy for gonococcal infection frequently changes. The current recommendations of the United States Public Health Service should be consulted.

In selecting a treatment regimen, the following factors should be kept in mind. 1) Patient preference—the patient's acceptance of therapy may influence his compliance with surveillance or his willingness to use the clinic for future infections. 2) Patient reliability—single-dose therapy is preferable for those who cannot be relied on to complete multiple-dose regimens. 3) Effectiveness of antibiotic—although other considerations may outweigh differences of a few percent in cure rates between different regimens, it is desirable to use a regimen with a cure rate of more than 90 percent. 4) Side effects—some side effects, such as penicillin allergy, involve specific individuals. Other side effects have a more general impact. For instance, tetracyclines should never be used for treating young children or pregnant women. In these cases, erythromycin may be used for the patient allergic to penicillin. 5) Effect on other diseases—the value of procaine penicillin against incubating syphilis, or of tetracycline against nongonococcal urethritis, may be relevant, depending on the prevalence of these diseases in any community. 6) Cost.

Procaine penicillin (4.8 million units) and probenecid (1 gm.) provide effective therapy for uncomplicated infections. Ampicillin (3.5 gm.) and probenecid (1 gm.) have been recommended for oral therapy. However, amoxycillin (3 gms) provides higher blood and urine levels than ampicillin[14] and may be preferred. Intramuscular spectinomycin (2 gm.) is a convenient, one-dose parenteral alternative for penicillin-allergic patients. Tetracycline (1.5 gm. orally, followed by 0.5 gm. at 6-hourly intervals for 4 days) also provides adequate therapy. Pharyngeal infections should be treated with procaine penicillin or tetracycline. Ampicillin and spectinomycin do not appear to be effective with this type of infection.

Early cases of PID may be treated on an outpatient basis with the procaine penicillin or ampicillin schedules for uncomplicated gonorrhea. This should be followed for 10 days by ampicillin (0.5 gm. 6-hourly). In more advanced cases, hospitalization and initial treatment with aqueous crystalline penicillin G (20 million units per day intravenously) is recommended. Following clinical improvement, the 10-day course of antibiotic is completed with ampicillin (0.5 gm. 6-hourly).

When nongonococcal PID is suspected, an aminoglycoside may be added to the above regimens. Alternatively, tetracycline (0.5 gm. 6-hourly, intravenously until improvement occurs, and then orally) may be administered for 10 days.

Disseminated gonococcal infection may be treated with antibiotic regimens similar to those used for PID. Immobilization of affected joints is indicated, and repeated aspiration and saline irrigation are recommended. Intraarticular administration of antibiotics is unnecessary.

Gonococcal conjunctivitis should be treated by conjunctival irrigation with penicillin, together with penicillin G given intravenously.

Nongonococcal Urethritis (NGU)[9]

Introduction

Urethral irritation and discharge may be physiological, due to semen or seminal components. It may be caused by mechanical or chemical irritation of the urinary tract, most commonly due to the introduction of chemicals or objects into the urethra, but also produced by manipulation of the genitalia. Concentration, and sometimes precipitation or crystallization, of the chemical constituents of the urine are also common causes of mild, transient urethritis. Urethritis may be the result of infection of the proximal urinary tract; e.g., cystitis or pyelonephritis. Irritation or discharge may be caused by infective urethritis, which may be bacterial, protozoal, metazoal, fungal, or viral.

Despite this array of possible causes, the present evidence suggests that the majority of sexually transmitted nongonococcal urethritis is caused by an infective organism, producing a fairly distinct clinical picture characterized by an incubation period, which is commonly 10–20 days; a variable discharge, usually mucopurulent in nature, and somewhat less copious than that generally encountered in acute gonorrhea; spontaneous remission in many cases, with possible improvement by placebo administration; and a clear-cut response to tetracycline (as opposed to placebo) in a large number of cases.

T-strain mycoplasma and *Chlamydia* are currently the two organisms of most interest in the etiology of nongonococcal urethritis. Evidence on mycoplasmas has been conflicting. While mycoplasmas have been isolated from over 50 percent of some groups of symptomatic men, a similar isolation rate has frequently been obtained from similarly promiscuous men who are asymptomatic.[15] *Chlamydia* have been more consistently isolated from a significantly higher proportion of symptomatic men than from asymptomatic controls.[16,17] Possibly 50 percent of NGU is due to *Chlamydia* infection.

Diagnosis

In the absence of an unequivocal causative agent, nongonococcal urethritis is diagnosed by demonstrating urethritis and excluding other venereal and nonvenereal causes. The following criteria should be used for diagnosis: a) the patient has dysuria and/or urethral discharge, b) the onset of symptoms is clearly related to sexual contact, c) an abundance of polymorphs in the urethral smear or urine sediment, d) the absence of intracellular diplococci in the urethral smear and the failure of gonococci to grow on Thayer-Martin medium.

The patient who demonstrates objective evidence of urethritis should be evaluated initially by preparing a Gram-stained smear of urethral secretions. If this shows Gram-negative intracellular diplococci, a presumptive diagnosis of gonorrhea is made and the patient treated accordingly. In the absence of diplococci the patient is treated for NGU. In the latter case, a culture is recommended to detect gonorrhea missed by the smear; a negative culture confirms the diagnosis of NGU.

When there are treatment failures with tetracycline, an examination of sex partners and examination of an anterior urethral smear for trichomonads may clarify the diagnosis. If trichomoniasis in the sex partner is the sole finding, epidemiologic treatment with flagyl is indicated.

Management

In the absence of specific laboratory diagnostic tests and with a vague clinical definition, it is necessary to establish and maintain firm diagnostic criteria. It is essential that an array of symptoms resulting from the patient's anxiety, physiological functions, or mechanical urethral irritation be clearly distinguished from the presentations of nongonococcal urethritis. These other conditions include spermatorrhea after defecation, minimal clear secretions after vigorous manipulation of the penis, and vague sensations of the genitalia unrelated to known symptomatic patterns and without any clinical evidence of pathology.

Tetrycycline is the drug of choice as being of proven value. It should be administered for 10 days (1.5 gm *stat.*, 0.5 gm *q.i.d.*). Penicillin and kanamycin, commonly used for gonorrhea, have little influence on the course of infection, nor is there evidence that other potent, broad-spectrum antibiotics are any more effective.

Relapses should be treated conservatively and with an optimistic approach. Mild hypersecretion of the genital glands may persist for months after infection. Minimal amounts of clear secretion, occurring intermittently and usually in the morning, in the absence of other symptoms should be accepted as a normal sequel of cured infection. When persisting symptoms, further diagnostic tests, and examination of sex partners suggest persistent NGU, a further course of tetracycline should be prescribed. The routine treatment of steady sex partners with tetracycline may reduce the recurrence rate.

Herpes Simplex Virus Infection (HSV)[18]

History

Clinicopathologic features of herpes simplex infection (cold or fever sores) have been known for many centuries, and clinical genital infection was first described over 200 years ago. In 1883 Unna suggested there was venereal transmission. The epidemiology of the disease has been clarified by the more recent detection of two antigenic variants, HSV–1 and HSV–2. The majority of HSV–2 infections are acquired during sexual contact or in association with parturition.

Clinicopathologic Aspects

Primary infection may occur on first exposure to either HSV–1 or HSV–2. As with most viral infections, this initial attack may be subclinical, but when symptoms do occur they are usually more severe than in recurrent attacks. The incubation period varies from 2 days to 20 days (with an average duration of 6 days). Neutralizing antibodies develop within 1–4 weeks of infection.

In individuals with impaired defense mechanisms (neonates, patients with severe burns, atopic eczema, malnutrition, severe systemic illness, or on immune suppressive therapy), the organism may be highly invasive. Primary viremia is followed by virus duplication in seeded body organs. Subsequent secondary viremia concludes with recovery or death of the patient.

In healthy individuals, however, viremia is unusual and infection is localized to superficial areas of skin or mucous membrane. The mouth is the most common site for primary HSV–1 infection (the lips are the most common site for recurrent infection). Lesions of the genitalia are usually produced by HSV–2. This primary infection may produce severe systemic disturbance with fever, headache, anorexia, and general malaise. The extensive local ulcerations of the genitalia and the affected lymph nodes may be exquisitely tender, particularly in women. Acute necrotic cervicitis may accompany the external genital lesions in women. It may also occur in the absence of such skin lesions. Unless complicated by secondary infection or locally applied medications, the lesions resolve spontaneously in 2–3 weeks. Although exogenous reinfection has been suggested as a mechanism of recurrent infection, HSV probably persists in a noninfectious form in the nerve tissue supplying the area of previous infection. Genital recurrence may be triggered by fever, menstruation, or emotional disturbances, but it often occurs without any obvious cause. Neutralizing antibody does not afford complete protection from clinical infection, nor is the antibody consistently changed by recurrent infection.

Epidemiology

Some 30–50 percent of the adults in higher socioeconomic groups (SEG) compared to 80–100 percent of the adults in lower SEG possess HSV antibodies. In the latter group, HSV–1 antibody tends to rise rapidly in the first 5 years of life and HSV–2 antibody after 14 years of age; HSV–2 antibody reaches a prevalence of 20–60 percent in adults in the lower SEG. By comparison, only 10 percent of adults in higher SEG, 3 percent of nuns, and almost 100 percent of older prostitutes have HSV–2 antibody.

Generally, herpes lesions below the waist are caused by HSV–2 and those above the waist by HSV–1. From 5 percent–10 percent of genital lesions may be caused by HSV–1, however, and HSV–2 may be isolated from oral lesions of those practicing fellatio or cunnilingus. Among individuals who have both oral and genital lesions, organisms of the same antigenic type (either 1 or 2) are often isolated from both sites, but any individual may have HSV–1 infection on one part of the body and HSV–2 infection on another.

Herpes virus is also transmitted by kissing and manual contact with infected areas. Although viral antibody transfer occurs *in utero,* transplacental transmission of the virus itself has not been conclusively demonstrated. The infant is frequently infected from maternal genital lesions after membrane rupture or during passage through the birth canal. Viral antibodies acquired *in utero* do not confer immunity from this infection. Probably one-half of those infected will die or be severely damaged.

Evidence on the relationship between HSV–2 infection and cervical carcinoma is conflicting.

Diagnosis

Many forms of herpes infection are readily identified on clinical grounds. The recurrent, grouped vesicular eruption on an erythematous base, with progressive crusting and resolution in about 7 days, offers little difficulty in diagnosis. When the infection involves mucous membrane or moist areas of the genitalia, laboratory examination may be required to confirm the diagnosis.

Cytologic examination of a smear (Tzank smear) from the lesion is the most convenient confirmatory aid. The smear should be made from the base of a previously unruptured vesicle, but a firm scraping from an erosion or ulcer can also be used. The slide is fixed with absolute alcohol for 1 minute and stained with Giemsa (or other hematologic) stain. Typical multinucleate giant cells characterize herpes infection. Ground glass intranuclear inclusions occur in the violet-staining nuclei.

Diagnosis can also be confirmed by isolation of herpes simplex virus in tissue culture. Culture samples should be taken from fresh lesions containing vesicular fluid and sent to the laboratory in Liebovitz-Emory or Stuart's medium. The virus may be typed by a plague appearance on tissue culture, cytopathic effect, or serologic techniques. Herpes simplex virus type 1 produces a pock of less than 0.5 mm. diameter after 3 days growth on egg chorioallantoic membane; HSV–2 usually produces a larger pock.

Management

The multitude of therapies used for herpes infections testifies to their limitations. A fatalistic attitude of nonintervention is to be deprecated, since the judicious use of available analgesic medications and both direct and indirect psychological support may greatly reduce the suffering of an otherwise stressful experience.

All lesions should be kept clean and free of infection by twice-daily soaks with dilute eusol or other chemical debriding agent. Local and systemic antibiotics may rarely be necessary to control infection, but steroid preparations should be avoided. Adequate analgesia with aspirin or codeine is an essential consideration in all severe attacks. In women, the entire infected area can be liberally coated with xylocaine or zinc oxide cream before urination if it is uncomfortable.

The photodynamic effect of certain natural dyes has been used in treatment, but the therapeutic efficacy of this technique is unproven, and some workers fear it may be oncogenic.

Patients should be counseled about the nature of the disease and its therapy. The association with cervical carcinoma[19] should be presented in perspective. The female patient or the wife of a male patient should be advised to have a routine Papanicolaou smear yearly.

Herpes genitalis presents a special problem when it is present in the pregnant woman who is near term. Delivery by Cesarean section should be considered.

The condom is probably the most effective means of preventing transmission of the disease during coitus.

Trichomoniasis[20]

History

The description of *Trichomonas vaginalis* by Donne in 1836 predated elaboration of the clinical entity "trichomoniasis" by Hohne in 1916. The pathogenicity of the organism was disputed for a long time, but few modern clinicians regard *T. vaginalis* as a commensal of the genital tract.

Clinicopathologic Aspects

In women, *T. vaginalis* produces primarily a vaginitis, but it may also colonize the urethra, paraurethral glands, and bladder. Although infection may be asymptomatic, symptoms often develop within 4–28 days of exposure. Classically, the acute illness has copious, frothy, yellow-green vaginal discharge, with reddened, friable vaginal mucosa. Edema of the vulva and ulceration from maceration may occur with more severe illness. In subacute and chronic infection there may be few symptoms or signs, except for exacerbations after some or all menstrual periods.

In men, *Trichomonas* may produce urethritis and prostatitis. Infection is usually asymptomatic, but itching of the urethra, mild dysuria, and variable urethral discharge sometimes occur. The contribution of *T. vaginalis* to the incidence of nongonococcal urethritis is highly variable from one environment to another.

Epidemiology

Sexual contact is responsible for transmission of the disease to most women and virtually all men. The prevalence of infection in women varies with locality, age, and race. The disease occurs mostly throughout the sexually active age groups but with less localization to the younger age groups (15–24) than occurs with the other venereal diseases. Infection appears less common in men, but it has frequently been detected in up to 70 percent of the male sex partners of infected women.

Diagnosis

Trichomonads are readily identified in wet preparations from vaginal or urethral discharge of symptomatic patients. A drop of discharge is mixed with a drop of normal saline and examined under light or darkfield illumination. *Trichomonas vaginalis* is intermediate in size between polymorphs and epithelial cells and is easily recognizable by its characteristic thrashing movements. The addition of 0.1 percent safranin may be helpful in detecting dead flagellates which stain an intense red, in contrast to living organisms, which remain unstained. Trichomonads can also be recognized in Giemsa-stained preparations by their blue-staining cytoplasm and the reddish-violet granulated nucleus. Asymptomatic or minimally symptomatic patients may have a few trichomonads, which are often attached to epithelial cells. These may be recognized by their morphology and their flagellar movements or movements of the undulating membrane. The most sensitive diagnostic aid is culture on Feinberg–Whittington or similar medium at 37°C for 48 hours, followed by microscopic examination for trichomonads.

In asymptomatic men, specimens for the foregoing tests should be obtained from early morning (preurination) urethral scraping. Examination of urine centrifugate or prostatic secretions may increase the yield of detected infections.

Management

Metronidazole 2 gm in a single dose given orally is the treatment of choice; it cures over 80 percent of infections. The patient should refrain from intercourse until his or her regular sex partners have received the same treatment. Because local preparations are ineffective alone and fail to speed the rate of improvement, they are rarely indicated except during pregnancy.

Metronidazole sometimes produces gastrointestinal disturbances that may be aggravated by smoking or alcohol ingestion. It may also produce darkening of the urine (due to azo-dye formation), but this is of no pathologic significance. Metronidazole passes into the fetal circulation and is present in the milk of the mother. Although no damaging effects have been noted in the newborn, it should not be used during the first trimester and only later in pregnancy when local preparations do not control symptoms.

Syphilis[21,22]

Introduction

Stokes defined syphilis as an infectious disease due to *Treponema pallidum*. It is of great chronicity, systemic from the outset, and capable of involving every structure of the body in its course. Syphilis may be distinguished on the one hand by florid manifestations and on the other by years of completely asymptomatic latency. The disease is transmissible to offspring in man and is treatable to the point of presumptive cure.

Controversy concerning the origins of the disease continues between those who consider that it was introduced to the Old World by Columbus and his sailors in 1493 and those who consider that the individual treponematoses (syphilis, yaws, bejel, pinta) have appeared as part of an evolutionary process in which clinical manifestations of treponemal disease are dictated by the general hygienic and socioeconomic status of any particular community. In any case, the name *syphilis* has its origins in a poem written by Frascatorius in 1530. The poem describes a swineherd, Syphilis, who acquired the disease.

In 1905, Schaudinn and Hoffman identified the causative organism of syphilis as *Treponema pallidum*, and Castellani identified *Treponema pertenue* as the causative organism of yaws. In 1938, Saenz identified *Treponema carateum*, the cause of pinta. Although these organisms are morphologically indistinguishable, they produce different lesions when inoculated into the hamster, and only *T. pallidum* invades the central nervous system.

A serologic test (WR) was first described by Wassermann in 1906, and in 1948 Nelson introduced a specific blood test for treponemal disease, the *Treponema Pallidum* Immobilization (TPI) test.

Clinical Features

Figure 7-1 outlines the clinical and serologic progression of syphilis. The course is variable, however, and over 50 percent of those infected will not have serious physical sequelae from their illness. Some of these infections will undergo spontaneous cure. Others will lapse into a period of latency until the host dies of some other cause.

Syphilis can be classified as congenital or acquired. Syphilis can be transmitted from an infected mother to the fetus. The sequelae to maternal infection include late abortion, a macerated stillbirth at term, an infected neonate with clinical signs of disease, an asymptomatic infected neonate, and a normal child. Both the likelihood of infection and the severity of manifestations in those infected are greater the earlier the stage of infection is in the mother. Notwithstanding this generalization, a normal infant may be born to an infected mother who may later give birth to an infected infant.

Acquired syphilis may be divided into a number of stages. The first of these is an incubation period of 9–90 days, but averaging 3 weeks. In the primary stage, a chancre develops at the site of inocula-

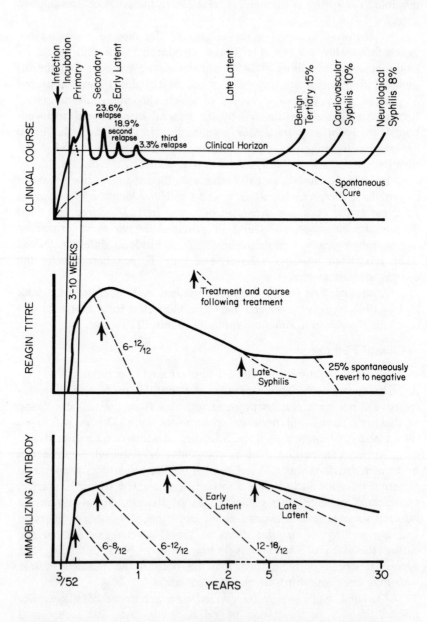

FIGURE 7-1 THE CLINICAL AND SEROLOGICAL COURSE OF SYPHILIS

tion. Probably less than 50 percent of primary chancres conform to the classical clinical presentation, but a solitary, painless, indurated ulcer, appearing 9–90 days following sexual contact, should always be investigated for syphilis. Acute genital ulcers that are indurated and painless are rarely caused by other organisms. Of course, chancres may be multiple and become painful should they become secondarily infected. Chancres may occur at any anatomic site, but are most common in the anogenital or oral regions. If untreated, the primary chancre will usually resolve spontaneously within 4 weeks.

The secondary stage of syphilis will appear 2–4 months after infection and will last several weeks. The more common manifestations of secondary syphilis include: systemic disturbance with fever, malaise, and generalized, nontender lymphadenopathy. There may be generalized macular or papulosquamous rash. This rash may mimic that produced by almost any other condition, but some features are helpful in making the diagnosis. The lesions are usually bilaterally symmetrical and rarely pruritic. Although vesiculobullous lesions may be seen in congenital syphilis, they never occur in adult-acquired syphilis. Pustular lesions are rare. Few other conditions produce similar lesions of the palms and soles. In later phases of the disease, when the rash develops papulosquamous features, confusion with psoriasis, tinea, and contact dermatitis may occur. There also may be oral lesions, mucous patches, or snail-track ulceration of the mouth and condylomata lata. These pale-colored, flat-topped papules occur in moist areas of the body, usually in the anogenital region. They are highly infectious. Another development may be circinate pigmented papular lesions, which commonly occur on the face. They have a sharp border and a central clear area. There may also be patchy, "moth-eaten" alopecia. This patchy alopecia may involve the beard, scalp, eyelashes, or the lateral third of the eyebrows.

A subclinical latent period follows the secondary stage; it may persist for the remainder of the patient's life. Positive serology provides the only indication that the patient is infected.

Finally there are late clinical manifestations, which may appear in up to 30 percent of infected individuals. These lesions may be cutaneous, visceral, cardiovascular, or neurologic.

Diagnosis

Detection of T. pallidum. The demonstration of *T. pallidum* either by darkfield microscopy or by fluorescent antibody (FA) methods provides unequivocal evidence of early syphilis. *Treponema pallidum* is a delicate, regular spiral organism, usually 7–12 μ in length and 0.2–0.25 μ wide. The organism moves slowly across the microscope field, may rotate around the long axis, and may exhibit mild concertina action or characteristic buckling or angulation.

Darkfield microscopy should be performed routinely on clear, serous fluid obtained from genital ulcers, nasal discharge, or the skin lesions of congenital syphilis, condyloma latum, or the other lesions of secondary syphilis. This method is unreliable for oral lesions, because naturally occurring saprophytes, particularly *Treponema microdentium,* are morphologically very similar to *Treponema pallidum.*

Serologic tests for syphilis. Serologic tests provide indirect evidence for syphilis, but are useful diagnostically when assessed in combination with a full clinical and epidemiologic knowledge of the patient. Serologic tests for syphilis may be conveniently divided into reagin tests (sometimes called standard or nontreponemal tests) and treponemal tests (sometimes called specific tests).

Reagin tests use purified cardiolipin combined with lecithin and cholesterol to detect an antibodylike substance usually present in the blood of syphilitics. These tests are relatively nonspecific, because reagin occasionally exists in the blood of individuals who do not have treponemal disease. Reagin may be detected by complement fixation, *e.g.,* Wassermann or Kolmer, or by flocculation techniques, *e.g.,* Kahn, VDRL. At present, the most commonly used reagin test is the venereal disease research laboratory (VDRL) slide test. This test is easily performed, is inexpensive, and can be readily quantitated by progressively diluting the serum.

The rapid plasma reagin (RPR) card test employs a modified VDRL antigen mixed with a suspension of carbon particles. In contrast to the VDRL, prior heating of serum is not necessary, and a microscope is not used for reading the results. This test is convenient where established laboratory facilities are not readily available. Some difficulty may be encountered in defining weak reactions, and titers may differ from the VDRL by one dilution (usually with the titer being higher when this occurs).

Treponemal tests include the Reiter protein complement fixation test (RPCFT), the *T. pallidum* immobilization (TPI) test, the fluorescent treponemal antibody-absorption (FTA-ABS test), and the *T. pallidum* hemagglutination (TPHA) test. The RPCFT uses a protein fraction derived from the Reiter treponeme, which shares a common antigen with *T. pallidum.* Although this test is simple, it is less specific

than other treponemal tests. It is therefore of limited value as a confirmatory test, although it may have a role in screening.

The TPI test detects antibodies by their power to immobilize active
T. pallidum. The test is cumbersome, requires a source of living treponemes, and is expensive. While the test may continue to have an important role in research, it is no longer warranted as a routine service
test. In cases that cannot be resolved by repeated VDRL titers, FTA–
ABS tests, and clinical and epidemiologic assessment, the diagnostic
or therapeutic significance of a TPI result, either positive or negative,
is uncertain. The FTA–ABS test is an indirect immunofluorescent procedure which uses dead *T. pallidum* as antigen. Crossreaction from
group antibodies is avoided by treating the patient's serum with sorbent,
a concentrated extract from nonpathogenic treponemes. The test may
be read negative, borderline, or 1+ through 4+. Following a borderline
or 1+ reading, the test should be repeated on a fresh serum specimen.
If the second test is 1+ or greater, the test is reported as reactive; if not,
it is reported as borderline. Most patients with a borderline FTA–ABS
do not have syphilis. The readings of 1+ to 4+ refer to the intensity of
fluorescence of the treponemes; the clinical significance of this variation
is unknown.

The FTA–ABS is currently the most useful treponemal test, but
it is not a simple test. It is performed poorly in some laboratories. The
best results can be expected if it is restricted to established laboratories,
carefully controlled, and performed regularly by the same experienced
technicians.

The FTA–ABS (IgM) test has been introduced for the diagnosis
of congenital syphilis. This test is based on the principle that IgM does
not cross the placenta; consequently, fetal treponemal IgM must be
manufactured by the fetus in response to infection, whereas IgG may
appear in fetal serum as a result of passive transfer from the mother.
Although initially promising, this test lacks both sensitivity and specificity. It requires further evaluation before it can be used routinely for
the diagnosis of congenital syphilis. Consequently, the diagnosis of congenital syphilis in the clinically normal neonate is best made presently
by detecting changes in the VDRL titer. The titer of passively trans-
ferred VDRL antibody usually declines rapidly within 3 months; therefore, a steady or rising titer suggests congenital infection.

The TPHA test uses the principle that red cells coated with ultra-
sonic lysate of *T. pallidum* agglutinate in the presence of specific treponemal antibody in the serum of syphilitics. This test can be quan-

titated (although the significance of different titers has not been established) and automated, and it has potential as either a screening or a confirmatory test. The antibody titer is not consistently influenced by treatment, and a reagin test must still be used for monitoring response to therapy.

False–positive serologic reactions. False–positive reagin tests occur in individuals who have reagin in their sera but do not have syphilis. This usually results from nontreponemal disease, but at times no cause can be found. In false–positive reactions, the VDRL titer is rarely higher than 1:4, but occasionally very high titers occur.

False–positive reactions may be acute or chronic. Acute reactions are of less than 6 months' duration and subside with their associated condition. The conditions implicated as causes of acute reactions include hepatitis, infectious mononucleosis, malaria, various viral conditions, and vaccination. Chronic reactions persist for more than 6 months. They have been associated with collagen diseases, leprosy, malignancy, narcotic addiction, and aging. Chronic false–positive reactions may be associated with a worse prognosis than true–positive reactions, and should be investigated accordingly.

False–positive findings in the FTA–ABS test may be due to collagen diseases, pregnancy, or other conditions. The TPHA may be false–positive in some individuals with cancer or diffuse skin diseases.

Performance of serologic tests. The performance of serologic tests is often described by their sensitivity and specificity (see Chapter 12), but the specificity of a test may vary with the population sampled. For instance, reagin tests may be fairly specific for screening a general population but are much less so when performed on individuals with diseases producing false-positive reactions. For this reason, there is a high incidence of false–positive reactions in underdeveloped communities due to the high prevalence of diseases producing these reactions. Table 7-2 compares the sensitivities of the major serologic tests at the different stages of syphilis. The FTA–ABS test is the first to become positive, is the most sensitive in primary syphilis, and is more sensitive than the TPI at all stages of the disease. The most adverse feature of the TPHA for screening purposes is its low sensitivity in primary syphilis. The VDRL is insensitive in late syphilis.

The specificity of the treponemal tests is more difficult to determine. When discordant results occur in the absence of supporting evidence, it is difficult to decide whether one test is false–positive, or the other false–negative. The TPI is probably more specific than the FTA–ABS, however, which is in turn more specific than the TPHA.

Use of serologic tests. The VDRL (or in special circumstances, the RPR) should be used as a standard screening test. The VDRL titer is also used to gauge the activity of disease and will give some indication of whether treatment or retreatment is required. Following therapy, the titer may continue to rise (sometimes a negative test becomes positive) for a short time before falling. A significant rise (two dilutions or a fourfold concentration) following this decline indicates relapse, and the patient should be retreated.

TABLE 7–2 SENSITIVITY OF VDRL, FTA–ABS AND TPHA DURING VARIOUS STAGES OF SYPHILIS[a]

Stage	% Reactive			
	FTA–ABS	TPI	VDRL	TPHA
Primary	86	53	76	77
Secondary	100	98	100	100
Early Latent	99	94	95	100
Late	97	93	70	100

[a] Rudolph AH, Duncan WC: Syphilis—diagnosis and treatment, Clin Obstet Gynecol 18: 163, 1975. Lensinski J, Krach J, Kadziewicz E: Specificity sensitivity and diagnostic value of the TPHA test, Br. J Vener Dis 50: 334, 1974

Treponemal tests give an indication of whether a patient has or has had syphilis but not whether he or she should be treated. Following a proven diagnosis of syphilis, further treponemal results are of no diagnostic or therapeutic significance unless previous seroreversal has been documented. Consequently, there are only two indications for performing an FTA–ABS test: a) an unexplained positive reagin test, or b) clinical suspicion of late syphilis.

It must be stressed that a positive reagin test is not explained merely by other illness of the patient. Common causes of false-positive reactions may coexist. The FTA–ABS is a good indicator of late syphilis (even when the VDRL is negative), because of the high prevalence of this condition in individuals who have suggestive clinical evidence of the disease.

Treatment

Penicillin remains the treatment of choice; a variety of regimens have been used. In contrast to the treatment of gonorrhea, the treatment of syphilis requires only a low level of antibiotic but requires it for a longer time; therefore, long-acting penicillins are generally used. For primary and secondary syphilis, one injection of 2.4 million units of benzathine penicillin is adequate. Alternatively, procaine penicillin may be administered daily for a period of 10–15 days. Where penicillin allergy exists, tetracycline (0.5 gm. *q.i.d* for 15 days) should be used. Erythromycin stearate (0.5 gm. *q.i.d*. for 15 days) may be used in pregnancy.

In late syphilis, penicillin therapy has less significance in the overall management of the patient. Although cardiovascular or neurologic damage may be irreversible, penicillin therapy may prevent further damage.

Cytomegalovirus Infection (CMV)[23]

Although Ribbert described cytomegalic inclusions in 1881, CMV infection, caused by a DNA virus of the herpes group, was first described as a clinical entity in 1956. The disease may be congenital or acquired. Either form may be covert or overt, with protean clinical manifestations.

Infection with cytomegaloviruses is worldwide, but transmission is imprecisely understood. Surveys in both the United States and England have demonstrated complement-fixing antibodies for CMV in over 50 percent of adults over 35. Approximately 50 percent of women in the childbearing age have serologic evidence of past or present infection. Clinical infection occurs in 3 percent–5 percent of pregnant women; congenital infection appears in 1 percent–3 percent of neonates. The prevalence of antibodies from acquired infection increases from about 4 percent in 5-year-old children to 15 percent–30 percent of 10-year-olds. It is almost universal in aggregates of children living in crowded conditions. Viruria has been found in 1 percent of children living at home and approximately 35 percent of institutionalized children.

Cytomegalovirus has been detected in semen and isolated from the cervices of over 13 percent of women suspected of having venereal infection.[24] It was significantly more common in women with a past history of gonococcal infection and reached a prevalence of 22.5 percent in the 20–24 age group. The quantitative contribution of sexual transmission to total disease dissemination has not been determined. Possibly CMV exists as two strains (as with HSV), and one strain is transmitted by sexual activity and the other by predominantly nonsexual activity.

The fetus may be infected in two different ways. There may be intrauterine transmission which produces the TORCH syndrome of deafness and other congenital abnormalities. Perinatal infection may be acquired during passage through the birth canal. This infection is less severe, but much more common than infection acquired *in utero*.

The infected child develops viruria in infancy but usually remains asymptomatic and suffers no obvious harm from infection. Detailed, long-term studies would be required to detect whether there is mild mental impairment or other subtle sequelae. This type of infection, if harmful, could presumably be prevented by cesarean-section delivery.

Clinical manifestations are influenced by host resistance. The manifestations are consequently more severe in congenital infection or infection of immunologically compromised individuals. Covert congenital infection may produce severe brain damage. Overt infection is characterized by jaundice, petechial rash, hepatosplenomegaly, choreoretinitis, and neurologic manifestations. Thrombocytopenia and hemolytic anemia are common. Acquired infection is usually asymptomatic, but it may produce hepatic dysfunction or respiratory symptoms. It may exist as a mild, chronic, febrile illness, with clinical features similar to infectious mononucleosis. The diagnosis of CMV may be confirmed by isolation of the virus from urine, throat or genital secretions, or demonstration of the pathognomonic haloed, "owl-eye" intranuclear inclusion bodies in smears stained with Giemsa or Papanicolaou stain. Changing titers of complement-fixing antibodies are indicative of infection; a titer of 1:32 or higher in the mother is supportive evidence for a diagnosis of congenital infection in neonates with the classical signs of the disease. The differential diagnosis includes toxoplasmosis, rubella, herpes simplex virus infection, and syphilis. There is no specific therapy of proven value.

Donovanosis (Granuloma Inguinale)[25]

History

Donovanosis was probably first described by McLeod in 1882. The causative organism, *Donovania* (alt. *Calymmatobacterium*) *granulomatis*, was discovered by Donovan in 1905.

Clinicopathologic Features

The primary lesion begins as an indurated nodule, which erodes to form a beefy, exuberant, granulomatous, heaped ulcer. This usually progresses slowly, often coalescing with adjacent lesions or forming new lesions by autoinoculation, particularly in the perineal region. Extensive acanthosis and dense dermal infiltrate, mainly plasma cells and histiocytes, occur. Some polymorphs are present in focal collections or scattered throughout the infiltrate, but lymphocytes are rare. The pronounced marginal epithelial proliferation may simulate early epitheliomatous change.

The infecting organisms invade mononuclear endothelial cells, reproduce, and mature within cystic spaces. The mature, encapsulated, ovoid bodies measure 1.5 × 0.7 microns and contain metachromatic bars which stain blue or black with Wright's stain. The pathognomonic feature of Donovanosis is this large, infected mononuclear cell, 25–90 microns in diameter, containing many intracytoplasmic cysts with deeply staining Donovan bodies. In chronic disease, healing and consequent fibrosis occurs concurrently with tissue destruction caused by the expanding lesion. Secondary infection often occurs, aggravating tissue destruction and residual scarring.

The genitalia are involved in 90 percent of cases, the inguinal region in 10 percent, the anal region in 5 percent–10 percent, and distant sites in 1 percent–5 percent. Lesions are limited to the genitalia in approximately 80 percent of cases and to the inguinal region in less than 5 percent. Unilateral and bilateral involvement are equally common. In the male, lesions most commonly occur on the prepuce or glans, and in the female on the labia. The most common distant sites infected are on the head (mouth, lips, throat, face), but involvement of the liver, thorax, and bones has also been reported.

Lesions become paler, less exuberant, and less friable a few days after the start of treatment. Shrinking of the lesions by peripheral epithelialization is evident after 7 days; total healing, except in grossly advanced cases, usually occurs within 3–5 weeks. Relapse frequently occurs, but it is more common if an antibiotic is not administered until the primary lesion has completely subsided.

Donovan bodies are usually no longer apparent in the smears after 5–10 days of treatment. If treatment is ceased at this stage, the lesion often continues to heal, but Donovan bodies may reappear in 7–10 days, and the lesion may become active again.

Diagnosis

The clinical presentation is highly suggestive of the diagnosis in most cases; however, diagnosis is readily confirmed by a stained crush preparation from the lesion. A piece of clean granulation tissue is spread finely and crushed between two glass slides, with the deep surface against the slide to be examined. The smear obtained is air dried and stained with Wright's or Giemsa's stain.

Donovan bodies appear as clusters of blue or black-staining organisms with a "safety-pin" appearance, due to bipolar chromatin condensation, in the cytoplasm of large mononuclear cells. Histologic examination of biopsied tissue is a less reliable diagnostic procedure, for the pathognomonic Donovan bodies are less frequently seen. Cultures on chick chorioallantoic membrane are not feasible routinely.

Treatment

While streptomycin and tetracyclines are often effective, resistance may develop. Gentamicin (I.M., 40 mg. *b.i.d.* for 14 days) and chloramphenicol (orally, 0.5 gm. *t.i.d.* until lesions heal) are probably the most effective drugs and cure most lesions within 3 weeks.

In any community, it is wise to use tetracyclines as first-line therapy, and then change progressively to streptomycin, chloramphenicol, and gentamicin if the efficacy of the current antibiotic wanes. If an antibiotic is effective, clinical response to treatment should be evident in 7 days.

Chancroid (Soft Sore)[25]

History

Chancroid was recognized as a clinical entity for centuries, but was not differentiated from syphilis until 1852, by Bassereau. The infective organism, *Haemophilus ducreyi*, was first isolated by Ducrey in 1889.

Clinicopathologic Aspects

The incubation period varies from 1–14 days, but it is usually less than 1 week. The lesions are much more common in uncircumcised men, apparently due to tissue maceration beneath the prepuce, which diminishes the normal integumental barrier to infection.

Lesions are usually confined to the genitalia. Entry of the organism is facilitated by preexisting abrasions. The most common sites are the internal surface of the prepuce, and frenulum in the male, and the labia, clitoris, fourchette, and vestibule in the female—sites which are most commonly traumatized during sexual contact.

A small papule, surrounded by a zone of erythema, first develops. It soon erodes to produce a sharply circumscribed, nonindurated ulcer with a granulating base. Multiple lesions may develop rapidly by autoinoculation; suppurative adenitis of the inguinal lymph nodes is common in untreated cases. Systemic spread does not occur. Superinfection may produce rapidly destructive lesions of the genitalia.

Although up to ten individual ulcers may occur, there are more usually one or two. Individual lesions vary from 1 mm. to 2 cm. in diameter, averaging 0.5 cm., but confluent, serpiginous ulceration of the coronal sulcus may encircle the penis.

Twenty-five to sixty percent of patients with chancroid develop the characteristic bubo. In over 70 percent of cases, it is unilateral, painful, unilocular, and spherical with marked redness of the overlying skin. Treatment begun shortly after the appearance of the lesion will abort the development of adenitis. Uneventful resolution usually occurs if treatment is commenced before the inguinal mass becomes fluctuant. If treatment is delayed, however, spontaneous rupture may occur, with resultant scarring and deformity. Treatment of the fluctuant bubo should include frequent, thorough aspirations (not incision) of the abscess, as well as systemic antibiotics.

Diagnosis

Hemophilus ducreyi is a slender, short (1–2 μ), Gram-negative bacillus with rounded ends. It has a tendency to form chains on culture, but in smears from primary lesions, it is most commonly observed in small clusters along strands of mucus.

The diagnosis of chancroid should only be made when presumptive evidence of this disease is obtained. Advice to make the diagnosis by exclusion of other conditions is unsatisfactory, since an array of nonspecific ulcerations will be included in this category and will cause confusion. All cases resembling chancroid should be investigated for syphilis, since the two diseases may coexist. Diagnosis may be made on any one of the following criteria: 1) culture of the organism, 2) detection of *H. ducreyi* as the sole organism in bubo aspirate, 3) smears showing *H. ducreyi* in chains or clumps along strands of mucus. Observation of organisms consistent with *H. ducreyi*, scattered among diverse other organisms, is an inadequate criterion for diagnosis. 4) A diagnosis of chancroid may be made if the clinical presentation suggests and any one of the following features is present: ragged, serpiginous ulceration of the coronal sulcus, severely erosive lesions, or the classical, unilateral bubo.

Treatment

Sulfisoxazole (1 gm. *q.i.d.* for 10–14 days) is the treatment of first choice. Tetracycline, alone or combined with sulfisoxazole, has also been used effectively. In some areas, particularly Southeast Asia, resistance to these drugs now occurs. These resistant cases should be treated with streptomycin or kanamycin (0.5 gm. *b.i.d.* for 10–14 days). These drugs should be used as first-choice treatment for erosive lesions and for all chancroidal lesions in environments where more than 10 percent of cases are resistant to sulfisoxazole. Intravenous cephalothin

(1 gm. at intervals of 6 hours) is usually effective in those cases re-sistant to kanamycin.

Local therapy is a helpful adjunct for subpreputial ulcers. The prepuce should remain retracted throughout the treatment and the ulcer-ative lesions cleaned thrice daily with a suitable debriding solution. Preputial retraction is contraindicated in the presence of preputial edema.

Lymphogranuloma Venereum (LGV)[25,26]

History

Wallace first described lymphogranuloma venereum in 1833, but a more comprehensive description was provided by Nicholas, Durand, and Favre in 1913. Gay-Prieto observed the causative organism in 1927.

Clinical Features

Lymphogranuloma venereum may be caused by several related, subgroup A *Chlamydia* organisms. There are three clinical phases of infection: inoculation and primary lesion, lymphatic dissemination with constitutional symptoms, and late complications. In any individual case, however, one or more of these phases may be absent or pass unnoticed.

A primary sore may appear on the genitalia, rectum, mouth, or, less commonly, at other sites within 3 days to 3 weeks after infection. The incubation period is usually 7–12 days. A primary genital lesion is noticed in about 30 percent of heterosexual men but less frequently in women. It is usually a small, painless vesicle or superficial, nonin-durated ulcer. It most commonly occurs on the coronal sulcus, prepuce, or glans in men, and on the fourchette, vagina, or cervix of women. Associated local or regional edema may produce phimosis or swelling of the labia. Rectal inoculation produces bloody anal discharge and tenesmus at first, followed by mucopurulent discharge, diarrhea, and cramps. Simultaneous inoculation into the mouth, genitalia, or other regions may occur. Oral infection without genital infection has been reported in a patient who practiced coitus and cunnilingus with all sex partners.

Primary lesions are followed in 7–30 days by adenopathy in the lymphatic drainage area of the inoculation site. The superficial inguinal nodes are involved when the primary lesion is on the penis, anal margin, clitoris, or upper vulva, but simultaneous involvement of the deep iliac lymph nodes occurs in over 75 percent of cases. Inoculation in the va-gina or cervix produces adenopathy in the deep iliac and anorectal nodes. Rectal inoculation produces adenopathy of the deep iliac, perirectal, and hypogastric nodes. Oral inoculation mostly produces submaxillary and cervical adenopathy, but following tonsillar inoculation, cases of supraclavicular and mediastinal lymphadenopathy and pericarditis have been recorded.

A sensation of stiffness and aching, followed by swelling of the inguinal region, is the first sign of infection for the majority of patients. Infection spreads to involve all nodes in the group, which become matted and attached to the overlying skin. The skin may have a characteristic purplish color. The nodes above and below Poupart's ligament are frequently involved. This produces the sign of the groove, a linear depression in the elongated, inflammatory mass. Inguinal adenopathy is unilateral in about 70 percent of cases. Adenopathy may subside spontaneously or proceed to the formation of abscesses, which rupture to produce chronic draining sinuses or fistulae.

Lymphatic spread is associated with variable constitutional symptoms. Mild fever frequently precedes adenopathy and lasts for several days. In other cases, high fever, sweating, and rigors occur. Malaise, nausea, and vomiting occur, particularly in those with high fever. Abdominal pain, urinary retention, and symptoms of cystitis are common when pelvic nodes are involved. Transitory myalgia and arthralgia are common, and erythematous skin lesions occasionally occur. Hepatomegaly, splenomegaly, nephropathy, meningismus, and phlebitis have been reported.

Common hematologic changes in this phase include mild anemia, leukocytosis, elevated sedimentation rate, hypolipidemia and hyperglobulinemia.

Diagnosis

The Frei skin test becomes positive 12–40 days after the appearance of the primary lesion and usually remains so for life; however, the test is less than 70 percent sensitive and is frequently negative, even in advanced stages of infection. It is also nonspecific and frequently reacts in individuals who have been infected with any of the chlamydial organisms.

The LGV complement fixation test (CFT) is 90 percent–95 percent sensitive, and becomes positive earlier than the Frei test (usually within 1–3 weeks). It is nonspecific, but it can be titrated, which enhances its value. However, neither the Frei Test nor the LGV–CFT is of great value alone. Certainly neither is of value as a screening test.

In the presence of the clinical syndrome, a fourfold rise in titer of the CFT is diagnostic. This test has usually risen to a stable titer by the time most patients present for diagnosis, and it may not decline significantly for several months.

Treatment

Early antibiotic therapy is important in reducing the morbidity of the disease, and treatment should never be withheld while awaiting laboratory proof of infection. Oral tetracycline is recommended (0.5 gm. at 6-hour intervals for at least 3 weeks). If pregnancy or idiosyncrasy preclude tetracycline, sulfisoxazole (4 gm. initially and 0.5 gm. every 6 hours) should be used. Fluctuant lymph nodes should be aspirated, but surgical intervention should otherwise be minimized.

The disease is characterized by remissions and exacerbations, and thorough surveillance is important. Full clinical assessment and LGV–CFT titer should be performed every 3 months for at least 1 year after cure. Antibiotic therapy should be recommenced immediately if there is evidence of reactivation.

Pediculosis Pubis

Introduction

Genital pediculosis is caused by *Phthirus pubis*, a blood-sucking louse 1–4 mm. long. These lice attach their eggs (nits) to pubic hairs. They rarely survive more than 24 hours off man. In contrast to head and body lice, they are mostly transmitted from person to person during sexual contact, though they may be spread *via* bedding, clothing, or nonsexual contact.

Pathology

The lice introduce saliva into the puncture site during feeding. This induces an erythematous papule within a few hours. Secondary bacterial infection may occur from subsequent scratching. There may be infiltration with lymphocytes and extravasation of erythrocytes. Residual pigmentation (so-called maculae cerulae) from this bleeding may be a prominent feature of long-standing infestation.

Clinical Features

Infestation with crab lice may be asymptomatic. The host may first become aware of the condition when he notices the parasite moving on the skin surface. Usually the patient seeks treatment for pubic itching, which may have resulted in abrasions that have become secondarily infected, causing further discomfort for the patient. Pigmented macules may mark the site of lice bites.

Diagnosis

The diagnosis is made by observing, with the aid of a hand lens, the presence of lice or their nits on the pubic hair.

Treatment

Benzyl benzoate (25 percent) or gamma benzene hexachloride (1 percent) lotion eradicate the lice. It is advisable to repeat treatment in 7–10 days (the incubation period of the lice), for some eggs may occasionally be missed with the initial application. Undergarments and bed linen should be laundered during the treatment period to destroy any stray lice. All sex partners should be examined and treated if they are infested.

Scabies

Introduction

Scabies is an infectious skin disease produced by the female mite of *Sarcoptes scabiei*, which burrows into the epidermis to feed and deposit her eggs.

The itch mite (*Acarus scabeie*) was described by Avenzoar in the twelfth century, but the etiologic relationship between scabies and *S. scabiei* was first demonstrated by Hebra in 1868.

The disease is associated with poor living conditions and has flourished in most war environments. Although adult mites can survive for a few days outside the host and while infection can occur from bedding or clothing, the disease is mostly transmitted from person to person by prolonged skin-to-skin contact. It can thus be spread by sexual contact. In communities where the disease is controlled or almost eradicated, outbreaks of infection often occur among sexually promiscuous groups. Sexual behavior becomes a significant epidemiologic feature. Species causing mange in animals are distinct from the human parasite, but they may cause clinical symptoms in man. Those who handle animals, particularly dogs, are the most prone to infection from this source.

Pathology

The gravid female burrows into the skin, depositing eggs and feces in the tortuous tunnel. The larvae hatch in 3–4 days and mature on the skin in 4–6 days, after which they mate, and the cycle is repeated. Sensitization producing itching develops in the host 1–3 months after infestation. There is infiltration of lymphocytes and eosinophils around the burrows, causing an eosinophilia of up to 15 percent. In individuals with a diminished or absent appreciation of itching (due to poor nutrition, illness, or psychological factors), Norwegian or crusted scabies may occur. Extensive ulceration and enormous numbers of parasites may accumulate under the hyperkeratotic plaques that develop.

Clinical Features

Symptoms develop when hypersensitivity has developed 1–3 months after initial infection. An itchy, erythematous, papular eruption appears. Secondary infection develops from the resultant excoriation. The eruption usually involves the axillae, waist, thighs, and flexures of arms and legs, but the crusts of Norwegian scabies may be located on any part of the body including the face and scalp. The itch of scabies is most noticeable when the host becomes warm, after a bath, or in bed. By contrast with lesions occurring elsewhere, those on the glans may not itch.

Diagnosis

In many cases, the diagnosis can be made on clinical grounds, but it sometimes requires confirmation by finding mites or eggs. Using a magnifying glass, an inhabited burrow between the fingers or around the wrist is located. The parasite may be extracted on a needle point and viewed under a microscope. Alternatively, a burrow top is shaved off, treated with 10 percent–20 percent potassium hydroxide, and the material viewed microscopically.

Treatment

Benzyl benzoate (25 percent) or gamma benzene hexachloride (1 percent) lotion produce almost universal cure when correctly applied. Following a bath, the preparation should be applied over the total body surface from the neck downward. To cover possible failure, the application should be repeated in one week. All intimate contacts should be examined and treated.

Corynebacterium Vaginale Infection[27,28]

Introduction

Although the organism has been known for decades, *Hemophilis vaginalis* was assigned as the etiologic agent of a specific vaginitis by Gardner and Dukes in 1955. In 1953, Zinneman and Turner suggested that the organism should be more appropriately named *Corynebacterium vaginale*, and this name is currently preferred.

Clinical Features

The majority of infected individuals are asymptomatic. When symptoms do occur, they are usually milder than commonly encountered in the vaginitides of acute trichomoniasis or moniliasis. Mild vulvovaginal irritation is experienced by 10 percent–40 percent of patients. Vaginal discharge is usually scanty, gray-colored, slightly offensive, and of uniform consistency, being mildly frothy in approximately 20 percent of cases. Marked redness and edema of the vagina occurs in about 10 percent of infections. A further 10 percent have minimal signs of inflammation.

Diagnosis

Microscopic examination of a wet mount presents a characteristic picture. Pus cells are rare, and lactobacilli are usually absent. The diagnostic feature is the "clue cell," an epithelial cell with a uniformly granulated appearance, due to the adherence of many *Corynebacteria* on the surface. Not all epithelial cells are affected in this manner.

In the Gram-stained smear, enormous numbers of small, Gram-negative bacilli are seen. A minority of other organisms occur, but lactobacilli are usually absent.

C. vaginale grows on modified Casman's blood agar as minute, smooth, glistening colonies. It is oxidase negative and ferments glucose and maltose but not lactose or sucrose.

Treatment

The most effective treatment is oral ampicillin (0.5 gm. *q.i.d.* for 8 days), but the use of antibiotics does not appear warranted for asymptomatic infection.

Condyloma Acuminatum[29]

History

Condyloma acuminatum has been known since antiquity, with clinical lesions described by the Greeks and Romans, but was only recognized as a distinct, separate entity (rather than a manifestation of other venereal infections) in the nineteenth century. Viral etiology was first suspected in the twentieth century, and venereal transmission was demonstrated in the 1950s. In the 1960s, the infecting agent was identified by electron microscopy as a papova virus. Condylomata acuminata are clinically and histologically distinct from verruca vulgaris, and genital wart antisera react only with genital warts. It is currently thought that condyloma acuminatum is caused by a mutant strain of the virus causing verruca vulgaris, with some immunologic cross-reactivity.

Pathology

Condylomata acuminata are luxuriant, fleshy growths. Histologically, there are deep rete pegs, containing well-differentiated, squamous epithelium with a fairly thick malpighian layer. The few mitoses seen are confined to the basal layer. Parakeratosis is usually seen, but hyperkeratosis is unusual, a feature which differentiates condyloma acuminatum from verruca vulgaris.

Clinical Features

The average incubation period is probably 2–3 months. Genital warts develop in over 50 percent of the sex partners of infected individuals and appear to be transmitted during sexual intercourse. The infectivity of genital warts decreases with their duration. In moist areas, the growths are fleshy and readily spread to adjacent areas. The exuberant forms most often involve the labia, introitus, and cervix in females, and the prepuce or urethra in males. In the female, condylomata often proliferate in pregnancy and may complicate labor by obstruction of the birth canal or hemorrhage due to trauma. Perianal and rectal warts in both sexes are often associated with rectal intercourse.

Diagnosis

Diagnostic aids are rarely necessary. Histologic examination may be required for unusual clinical presentations, however.

Treatment

Podophyllin (20 percent–25 percent in tincture of benzoin compound) may be used for small lesions but is not recommended for large lesions. Contact with adjacent normal tissues in moist regions often produces severe inflammation, necrosis, and pain; extreme care must be used if podophyllin is applied there. Podophyllin is contraindicated in pregnancy, due to potential toxicity to the mother and fetus.

Surgical management by excision and cautery is the treatment of choice for large condylomata, since the tissue necrosis from podophyllin may cause severe cellulitis. Depending on the number and site of the lesions, local or general anesthetic is required. Careful cryosurgery is a useful measure that obviates the need for anesthesia, but it is mainly applicable to sessile lesions. Lesions involving the urinary meatus or urethra should be referred to a urologist for specialist management.

For resistant cases or in massive genital involvement, autogenous vaccine therapy may have a role. The vaccine is prepared from excised condylomata and administered as 6 weekly injections of 0.5 ml.[30] There is usually evidence of response in 3–4 weeks.

Condylomata should be treated conservatively during pregnancy, unless they are likely to cause complications during delivery. Recurrence is common during this period, and spontaneous resolution often occurs at the end of pregnancy.

Molluscum Contagiosum

History

Molluscum contagiosum was first described as a clinical entity by Bateman in 1814. Henderson and Paterson described the characteristic cellular inclusions in 1841.

Pathology

The infective pox (DNA) virus infects most of the epidermal cells in an area of epithelium spanning several rete ridges. Epithelial proliferation produces pear-shaped lobules which slant toward the center of the lesion to produce a cup-shaped crater containing loosely adherent, infected epithelial cells. The cytoplasm of each infected cell is largely replaced by the molluscum contagiosum inclusion body. This central mass constitutes the pealike core of the lesion.

Epidemiology

The distribution of molluscum contagiosum is worldwide, but is most common in underdeveloped countries, with a prevalence of over 20 percent in some South Pacific communities. This suggests that poor hygiene and crowded living conditions may contribute to dissemination.

Although the disease occurs mostly in children, where it involves the trunk and extremities, adult infection involving the pubes, genitalia, and inner thighs is becoming more common. There is little doubt that this latter syndrome results from sexual contact, and similar lesions are sometimes found in sexual partners. The long incubation period of the disease explains the relative infrequence of partner infection in promiscuous individuals.

Clinical Features

The incubation period is probably 2–3 months. When occurring on the limbs or trunk, molluscum contagiosum appears as characteristic, pearly, spherical papules, 3–5 mm. in diameter, with central umbilication. Lesions may occur singly, but usually from 10–30 of them are found. In adults, the lesions are often confined to the lower abdominal wall, pubes, inner thighs, and genitalia. These are often larger and fewer in number than lesions elsewhere.

Diagnosis

The distribution, appearance, and characteristic central umbilication enable clinical diagnosis in most cases. In doubtful cases, diagnosis may be confirmed by microscopic examination of the core material. This can be crushed and examined unstained for the typical, large, cytoplasmic inclusion bodies.

Management

Spontaneous resolution is usual within 2 years. Often it occurs much sooner. Due to the benign nature of the lesion, treatment depends on the wishes of the patient. The treatment of choice is incision of the fine capsule with a scalpel blade or 18-gauge needle, and extrusion of the central core. This is a nearly painless procedure, bleeding is usually negligible, and the residual skin tags gradually resolve.

Candidiasis[31]

Introduction

Although not a venereal disease, candidiasis is often seen in venereal disease clinics; candidiasis and trichomoniasis together are responsible for most cases of vaginal infection.

Candida albicans is a dimorphous fungus which exists mainly as a saprophyte of man. It is isolated from the mouth, vagina, or intestine of healthy individuals at the rate of 25 percent–50 percent at each site, but most individuals probably carry the fungus at some time at some site.

The change from saprophytic to pathogenic status results from generally diminished host resistance or from factors which change the environment at some local site, enabling *Candida* to proliferate. The most important factors involved include the following.

Heat and moisture. Moisture is a prerequisite for the development of cutaneous candidiasis. Under experimental conditions, infection was established only when an occlusive dressing was placed over the inoculation site. Cutaneous candidiasis is more common in the tropics and among certain occupational groups whose skin is subject to moisture or heat.

Estrogen and progesterone levels. Vaginal candidiasis, in particular, is more common in women at periods of high estrogen and high progesterone levels. Thus, it predominates premenstrually, late in pregnancy, or in those taking oral contraceptives.

Broad-spectrum antibiotics.   Ingestion of tetracycline, ampicillin, or other broad-spectrum antibiotics is often associated with symptomatic vaginitis. The antibiotic may act directly by removing lactobacilli or other bacteria from the normal flora, or alternatively by increasing the glycogen content or pH of vaginal secretions.

Diabetes.   The increased risk of recurrent yeast infection in diabetics presumably results from the increased glucose substrate in blood, saliva, and other body fluids.

Steroids.   Steroids may favor infection by increasing glucose levels or reducing the immune response.

Systemic disease.   Candidiasis, particularly systemic infection, sometimes results from malignancy, chronic infectious diseases, or malnutrition.

Parturition.   Neonates are particularly susceptible to oral or cutaneous infection, which is often transmitted from the vagina during birth.

Although candidiasis is rarely transmitted by sexual contact, the saprophytic organism may be passed from one person to another, or from one site to another on the same person, during sexual activity. In most cases, this passage is associated with disease only if there is some predisposing factor in the host. In the male, balanitis may result if yeast from the vagina is deposited on a moist or macerated glans (usually in the uncircumcised). Probably the greatest risk for vaginal infection results from inoculation, *via* the penis or fingers of her partner, with yeast from the woman's own intestinal tract.

Clinical Features

Candida may produce an array of disease entities, including congenital cutaneous infection, gastrointestinal infection, paronychia, intertrigo, folliculitis, cheilitis, and disseminated disease. Vaginitis and balanitis are the two entities most frequently encountered in venereology.

Classically, *Candida* vaginitis produces a marked pruritis and thick, white, curdy, adherent discharge. Dyspareunia is common. These symptoms are usually worse premenstrually or during pregnancy or are related to oral contraceptives, steroids, antibiotics, or diabetes. Examination usually reveals excoriation and edema of the vulva, reddening of the vagina, and white, granular discharge.

Balanitis is a generalized inflammation of the glans penis from which *Candida* and a variety of bacteria can usually be isolated. However, the etiologic role of these organisms is uncertain.

Diagnosis

A vaginal smear may either be treated with a drop of 15 percent–20 percent potassium hydroxide and examined as a wet preparation, or be air dried, fixed with alcohol, and stained with Giemsa, Wright, methylene blue, or Gram stain. The yeast form of *Candida* appears as clusters of sperical, densely staining blastospores, 1–2 μ in diameter. In active disease, wide, irregular mycelial forms should also be seen. In clinical practice there is no reason to culture *Candida* from the glans penis or vagina.

Treatment

The aim of treatment is to alleviate existing symptoms and to maintain the patient as symptomfree as practicable. In managing vaginitis, the physician assesses the environmental/host factors influencing infection, provides anticandidal medication as required, and counsels the patient about the disease. Only the patient can decide her precise management, since this may be influenced by the subjective physical or psychological impact of the disease, her contraceptive choice, and other behavioral preferences.

Nystatin suppositories, inserted each night for 2–3 weeks, are usually effective in the acute attack. Amphotericin B suppositories are not more effective. Oral nystatin may temporarily remove *Candida* from the intestine but is not absorbed. It is only indicated in selected cases of severe recurrent vaginitis.

The most important component of the management of balanitis is to keep the inflamed area clean and dry. In the absence of preputial edema, the prepuce should be retracted throughout therapy. Lotions containing nystatin or suitable antibiotics may be useful in severe cases where specific organisms have been identified.

Chapter Eight

Environmental and Individual Factors

Environmental Stress

"The circumstances which led to promiscuity would certainly have produced severe emotional disturbance in most people."[1]

Most societies attempt to monitor sexual behavior within strictly defined barriers. Despite rigid norms within individual societies, patterns of sexual behavior are diverse, both between different cultures and in the degree to which these patterns conform to society's standards.[2,3,4] While sociosexual standards are resistant to sudden change, the sexual behavior of the individual may change suddenly and dramatically in response to personal or environmental stress.

Such stress may occur in any situation where the individual is isolated, physically or psychologically, from the stable community on which he has relied for balanced social expression. This isolation may be due to a personally chosen profession, *e.g.*, soldiers, seamen, commercial travelers. It may also be due to measures such as institutionalization imposed by society or to social turmoil, such as war, quite beyond the control of the individual. Superimposed on these broader features of the environment, boredom, loneliness, conflict with superiors or peers, low job satisfaction, or difficulties in interpersonal relationships may result in maladjustment.[5]

Reports from many war environments provide a clear picture of the impact of stress on sexual behavior and its sequelae. Prebble[6] attributes the high incidence of venereal disease in wartime to the associated environmental upheaval. In Indian troops the incidence of venereal disease was very low in peacetime. Recruits were specially selected, given regular leave, and were frequently stationed near their homes. With the onset of war, these conditions changed. The troops had more money, they were isolated from their homes, and they came into close contact with heavily infected prostitutes—consequently venereal disease was common.

With continued separation from family and the prolonged tensions of war, the individual tends to assume a different outlook toward the standards and taboos he has previously accepted. Wessel and Pinck[5] suggest this "leads to the attitude that it is 'culturally normal' to seek occasional sexual outlets." Stouffer describes the same phenomenon:

> For men in combat. . . . under great anxiety and insecurity, men tend to lose many of their usual long term perspectives. At the same time their need for emotional reassurance was especially great; faced with the immediate possibility of personal annihilation amid the vast impersonal destruction of war, hedonistic drives and socially derived needs combined to make sexual deprivation a major stress.[7]

This psychological pressure is expressed, somewhat emotionally, by Butler:

> the soldier involved in the heat and circumstance of "battle, murder and sudden death" in particular in a war of attrition, must be regarded differently from the same man in peace . . . sordid task begets sordid passions . . . the artificial bars that in man's social life tend to restrain or sublimate the "sex-lust" are also thrown down.[8]

While physical danger and deprivation have an undoubted psychological impact on the soldier, boredom, loneliness, inactivity, low job satisfaction, hostility to military regimentation, and lack of recreational facilities are the environmental features that are notorious for fostering sexual escapism and its sequelae.[5]

> They often spent long period of enforced idleness in which the intense boredom of having no goals for activity was intermingled with anticipatory anxiety of waiting for further combat. . . . Monotony and boredom may appear to have been trivial compared with the shocks of attack, but they did take a psychological toll of more than negligible importance.[7]

The impact of inactivity on venereal infection is well documented. Greenberg[9] states the experience of the United States: "Venereal disease was a problem particularly during periods when the troops were

not actively campaigning in the field, and in garrison troops at all times."
Venereal disease was a major problem among British troops in the 2
years following the Armistice and demobilization in 1918. "During this
period, a huge army was comparatively idle and as could be expected,
the prevalence of V.D. increased rapidly."[10] Ratcliffe[11] presents the
same view from Southeast Asia: "the VD incidence rate is directly and
conversely related to the degree of active employment within a unit and
consequently prolonged unemployment or employment in apparently
pointless tasks will be reflected by an increase in venereal disease."
Australian experience has been similar: "With this quiet phase of garrison duty, we were soon faced with the problem that has endangered
armies over the centuries, the venereal diseases."[12] In World War I,
it was noted that the Australian and British troops had a similar incidence of VD when they were in France; in Britain the Australian rate
was four times as great. Venereal disease proved to be a disease of leave
or leisure.[8] Wittkower and Cowan[1] attribute the disparity of venereal
disease incidence in a field division and static unit (two and a half times
as great as in the former) to the "browning off" which inevitably accom-
panies inactivity.

There can be no doubting the severity of stress that causes soldiers
to behave in a manner they would not have envisaged when society is
more stable. "In men who could be classed as good soldiers the circumstances which had led to promiscuity would certainly have produced
severe emotional disturbance in most people."[1] This environmental influence is clearly illustrated in a study by Ehrmann[13] in which 302 war
veterans were compared with 274 nonveterans. Although the behavior
of the two groups was similar in a stable society (37 percent of the
veterans and 40 percent of the nonveterans were currently having intercourse), the impact of foreign service produced a much higher intercourse rate in the veterans. Intercourse had been experienced by 80
percent of the veterans who had served more than one year overseas
compared to 57 percent of nonveterans. Furthermore, many of the veterans had experienced intercourse only during the period in which they
were separated from their stable homeland society.

Gardner[14] has suggested that wartime conditions tend to foster
a spurious acceleration of maturity. The youth leaves home, is trained
to defend his country, and is suddenly thrust into a life-and-death situation. He is introduced to all the physical stresses of manhood while still
a youth emotionally. The expression of aggression in wartime may
heighten or augment other instinctual urges such as the sex drive. There
is an intensification of an inner drive at a time when there is lessened
external control.

Also, the army emphasizes virility, the markers of which are high alcohol intake, abnormal aggression, and profanity.[15] There may be powerful group sanctions favoring sexual relations with prostitutes, making abstention difficult.[16]

Due to the commercial potential of sexual activity, entrepreneurs rarely overlook likely markets. Prostitute opportunism and seduction, at both a subtle and blatant level, make a considerable contribution to promiscuity and venereal disease in stressful environments. Prostitutes flock to areas providing a market for their services—around army camps, hotels, wharves, etc. Competition is keen, and there are few rewards for the hesitant. Active touting, body contact, or explicit sexual stimulation may be utilized to encourage the reluctant client. Hotels, holiday resorts, and convention gatherings often provide sexual partners as part of a general service. Where groups of individuals are involved, there may be strong peer pressures to indulge in sexual activity. Against this background, sexual participation and exposure to venereal infection is not so much a result of succumbing to sexual desire as an inability to withstand the pressures to participate.

When this occurs, the individual may indulge in atypical behavior which he later regrets. Guilt and shame are likely to be more severe and occur more commonly than in individuals who routinely behave in a similar manner. Subsequent venereal infection, particularly where sexual relations with the marital partner have already resumed, aggravates any psychological distress.

In addition to the obvious external pressures of certain environmental situations, there is a substantial subjective component to the stress experienced by the individual. The many environmental pressures operating tend to have a cumulative effect. The final precipitant of venereal exposure may be relatively minor. This may be a trivial domestic argument, disagreement with workmates or superiors, or a minor physical illness. For men absent from their wives poor accommodation, monotonous diet, lack of recreational facilities, and inadequate postal deliveries or communication facilities contribute to individual dissatisfaction. Attention to these details, discarded as insignificant by some authorities, is likely to facilitate general social adjustment and minimize undesirable sequelae.

Individual Factors

"There is, of course, no such thing as an average venereal disease patient. He is a statistical artifact."[17] Although environmental stress is undoubtedly a potent influence on sexual behavior and its sequelae, personal factors affect the manner in which the individual adjusts to this stress. In stable environments, a small proportion of the population often provides a large proportion of venereal disease. To give some examples, over 50 percent of male gonorrhea patients in a London clinic had had previous infections. This proportion increased from 54.8 percent in 1953–1955 to 59.2 percent in 1959–1961. In this period the average number of previous attacks rose from 1.6 to 3.1. In 1959–1961, 10.3 percent of West Indians (who had experienced seven or more infections) provided 48.3 percent of infections. Of 1,000 patients with gonorrhea in the United States, 80 percent had previous infections, and 26 percent returned with new infection within 6 months.[18] In Los Angeles, of 209 males admitted with gonorrhea, 133 (65 percent) had had one or more previous infections. Nearly half of these were reinfected within 30 days following treatment.[19] In Greenland, 49 percent of males and 68 percent of female patients had three or more previous attacks.[20]

When environmental stress induces promiscuity in a larger proportion of the population, the physical sequel of this behavior, venereal disease, is shared more evenly. Among Canadian soldiers who were studied, 86 percent of the patients presented with their first infection. This included 5 percent who were infected at their first intercourse. Fourteen percent had had previous infections.[1] A survey of 3301 American personnel in Korea revealed that 863 (28 percent) had acquired VD while in Korea. Of these, 75 percent had one infection, 17 percent two, 5 percent three, 2 percent four, and 1 percent had between five and seven infections.[9] Among Australian soldiers in Vietnam, 65 percent had intercourse with prostitutes, and 27 percent of these men acquired venereal disease. Of the 27 percent, over 72 percent were infected only once. The pattern of venereal disease is similar following the social upheaval consequent to urban migration in developing countries. In New Guinea only 6 percent of military patients and 15 percent of civilian venereal disease patients had been infected previously.[21]

Although the existence of these high-risk groups, particularly in stable societies, has been demonstrated, definition of the sociological parameters responsible for this phenomenon is more difficult. Because of pronounced sampling bias and absence of controls, the findings of many studies relating to these characteristics are virtually meaningless. Secondly, these sociological parameters are often interrelated. Analyzing their influence independently may be misleading, even statistically unjustifiable. When more fundamental or integrated qualities such as personality or socioeconomic status are introduced, problems of definition and measurement arise. Despite these difficulties, examination of the individual factors associated with venereal infection is still of value in considering control policies.

Race

Many reports have demonstrated a much higher infection rate in black than in white Americans. The incidence of VD in black soldiers in World War II was several times higher than in whites both at home and abroad.[7] In Italy in 1945, 54 percent of blacks had been infected at some time, and 21 percent had been infected while overseas. The corresponding figures were 15 percent and 8 percent for whites. Blacks contributed 15 percent to the theater strength but 36 percent to the VD incidence.

Two main factors operated to produce this pattern. First of all, blacks had intercourse more frequently; about one-third more blacks than whites reported intercourse while in the theater. Participants had intercourse two or three times a month compared with once or twice for whites. Secondly, blacks associated with a class of woman more likely to have VD. The VD rate was 7/1000 contacts for blacks and 4/1000 contacts for whites. Brody[22] also demonstrated this marked difference between the two racial groups of soldiers. Civilian studies have shown the same trend, even when allowance has been made for differences in social class.[23-25]

In British West Africa during World War II, the venereal disease rate among European troops varied from 2.2 percent *per annum* in Gambia, 4.6 percent in Sierra Leone, 8.5 percent in the Gold Coast to 10 percent in Nigeria, although in some units it reached 40 percent *per annum*. Among African troops, however, the rate was 12 percent in Gambia, 28 percent in Sierra Leone, 50 percent in the Gold Coast, and over 60 percent in Nigeria.[26]

In New Zealand, Maoris contributed 19 percent of the gonorrhea reported in Christchurch, although they formed only 1 percent of the local population.[27] In Australia, aborigines contribute disproportionately to syphilitic infections.

Many factors, including behavior, attitudes, socioeconomic status, education, and availability of medical services, obviously contribute to this disparity in infection rates between different racial groups. The main significance of the differences is in identifying high-risk groups and providing an indication of the yield from screening surveys.

Age

High infection rates tend to occur in younger age groups. In 1971 in the United States the syphilis rates per 100,000 for the 15–19, 20–24, and over-50 age groups were 19.8, 41.3, and 1.8, respectively. The gonorrhea rates in Canada for the same year for the 15–19 and 20–24 age groups were 20.4 and 36.9. Similar patterns were noted in many other countries.[28] Among Australian troops in Vietnam, 84 percent of soldiers under 21 compared to 58 percent of those over 30 had intercourse in the war zone. This was reflected in a disproportionate contribution to the venereal disease rate by those under 21 (25 percent of VD patients compared with 13.7 percent of controls). Those over 30 were underrepresented (3 percent of VD patients compared with 8.4 percent of controls).[29]

Despite these findings, the reverse relationship has also been observed.[30] In one military study, 28 percent of VD patients compared to 43 percent of the controls were younger than 22.[31] Other investigators have not detected any relationship between age and risk of infection.[32,33]

A higher infection rate in younger age groups may be expected because this is the most sexually active section of the population. It is possibly of more interest to know whether these groups have a higher infection rate per contact, but this information is not readily obtainable. The important feature is that the majority of venereal disease patients are young people under 30. The therapeutic approach must be tailored to suit this age group. This group has decidedly different attitudes, standards, and behavioral patterns than older groups. The venereologist who has limited understanding and poor rapport with these young people must expect diminished cooperation from his patients and consequent inadequate management of venereal disease.

Marital Status

The influence of marital status depends on whether the marital partners are living together or are temporarily or permanently separated. In a normal stable environment, venereal disease is usually less common among the married, who are generally less promiscuous than their single counterparts. One study showed that infection was more common among divorced, separated, and widowed persons than among either the married or single.[24] Certainly severe marital upheaval or separation is a particularly critical period. Both partners are vulnerable to erratic and often quite atypical sexual behavior that renders them susceptible to venereal infection. In response to the loneliness and intense emotional turmoil often associated with separation, the individual may seek solace in a sexual relationship with almost any casual acquaintance. The psychological sequelae from this tarnished moral self-image may be as disturbing as any physical harm, particularly when marital reunion and resumption of normal activity follow a brief separation. The medical attendance of both partners with venereal infection in such a situation provides the venereologist with the challenging task of minimizing the impact of the physical and psychological sequelae of the transient disruption and aiding the marital repair. If instead the venereologist sees this situation as merely two more cases of VD requiring diagnosis and treatment, his management of the two patients is inadequate. This is the real significance of marital status in the management of venereal disease. Those who are married or those with more permanent partners are more likely to suffer complex social disruption as a consequence of their infection. The alleviation of the problems of this disruption is an inalienable component of their proper management.

The influence of marriage, both on infection and on the sequelae of this infection, differs markedly between different racial groups. In one study it was observed that while marriage appeared to deter infection among whites it had no significant influence on black males.[30] A similar difference was noted between black and white American soldiers.[22]

When men are separated from their wives, the marital bond usually has little influence on their behavior, although married men show a higher resistance to venereal infection.[1,22,31,34] However, marriage may still have some influence on behavior as typified by the findings on Australian troops in Vietnam.[29] Almost 70 percent of the single and 51 percent of the married troops had intercourse with Vietnamese prostitutes. This was reflected by a disproportionate contribution to the percentage of venereal disease patients by single unattached soldiers (53 percent of VD patients compared to 36.4 percent of controls: compared to 20.5 percent and 27.4 percent, respectively, for married soldiers).

Education

Education has a dominant influence on susceptibility to venereal infection. An inverse relationship between these two parameters has been detected in many studies both military and civilian.[7,17,22,24,31,35-37]

While there is usually a gradually decreasing infection rate with increasing education, the most dramatic reduction occurs among those with tertiary or university education. This group has both a reduced promiscuous outlet and an even greater reduction in their VD contribution. The better-educated individual is able to derive satisfaction from a wide array of activities and is less dependent on sexual outlet in periods of stress. In selecting a sexual partner he is more discriminating and tends to establish a more stable relationship than his less-educated counterpart. There is also a direct relationship between education and fellatio, masturbation, and other sexual practices associated with a reduced risk of infection. Prophlaxis is also utilized more commonly by this group.

Intelligence

Although it has been suggested that promiscuity and venereal disease are associated with less than average intelligence,[17,22] this is debatable for two reasons: assessment of intelligence is itself controversial, and many studies on venereal disease patients do not include adequate controls for evaluating this factor. The high incidence of low intelligence in many infected patients[38-40] may merely reflect the intelligence of the micropopulation from which they were sampled. Ahrenfeldt[41] minimized both these limitations by assessing controls and VD patients among British soldiers in Germany on a six-point army intelligence scale. The proportion of VD patients in the lowest two intelligence gradings were 33.5 percent and 6.5 percent; the corresponding proportions of controls were 21.0 percent and 4.8 percent.

It is doubtful if low intelligence is a significant determinant of venereal infection. Even when an association between these two parameters is demonstrated, any consequent epidemiologic implications are not obvious.

Socioeconomic Status

Many studies have suggested an inverse relationship between social status and venereal infection.[24,30,36,42,43] Conversion of the broad concept of socioeconomic status into valid quantifiable and scalable parameters is beset with many difficulties. Education, income, occupation, and parental occupation are components of social status, but for many individuals these criteria give contradictory indications of allocation on a single scale. Unequivocal classification and stratification of occupation alone is virtually impossible. In view of these difficulties, as well as the limited application of data relating socioeconomic status to venereal infection, it is more appropriate to confine investigation to the simpler, individual components of this characteristic.

Parental Influence

Because of its unique role in providing the major environmental background during the formative years, the parental home is a key factor in the social adjustment of the individual. Deficiencies in this influence are reflected by an array of antisocial sequelae of which venereal disease may be just one manifestation. Complete disruption of the parental home is the most obvious evidence of discord and is a common feature in the background of venereal disease patients.[36,39,44-46] More subtle defects in either the home environment or parent/child relationships may have a marked effect on social adjustment.

Abnormal childhood environment (emotional instability, separation, or divorce of parents) has been implicated as a contributing factor in venereal infection (36 percent of VD patients and 18 percent of controls).[31] A strict upbringing with an unsatisfactory parental attitude to sex has also been blamed (83 percent of VD patients and 48 percent of controls).[37]

The association of venereal infection with family size reflects a more complex influence of the parental home. Singh[37] found 56 percent of VD patients compared to 42 percent of controls came from families of more than four children. In another study, 12 percent of patients compared to 4 percent of controls came from families of four or more children.[47] The critical family size of four children is emphasized by the findings on Australian troops in Vietnam. The intercourse rates with prostitutes were 55.5 percent and 54 percent for those with one and two siblings, respectively. These rates were 79 percent, 65 percent, and 73 percent for those with three, four, and more than four siblings, respectively. Of even more significance was the relationship of parental approval of promiscuity and venereal infection to family size. Although the most common paternal response anticipated by soldiers was indifference (42.5 percent), maternal disapproval was envisaged by a majority (83 percent). Among those from families of more than five children, maternal approval (72 percent) was much more common than disapproval (22 percent). In large families it is possible that maternal ties are weaker than in small families. Promiscuity may be encouraged by any conditions which weaken maternal influence, either partially or completely. It might be anticipated also that loss of a mother might be a significant factor in encouraging promiscuous behavior in a home environment.

Associated Crime

A marked association has been noted between venereal infection and criminal offences—juvenile, adult, and military.[1,22,48,49] Among Australian soldiers, intercourse with prostitutes was experienced more commonly by those convicted of civilian crime (80 percent to 59 percent of controls) and by those with multiple military convictions (71 percent to 61 percent of controls). Those with multiple military charges contributed 42 percent of the venereal disease patients compared to 21 percent of the controls.

There is little doubt that venereal infection and crime are not causally related but are both manifestations of general social maladjustment. It has been suggested that certain types of personality may predispose to these sequelae.[50] It is clear, however, that both promiscuity and venereal infection are more common in those with criminal convictions. Moreover, these individuals are often poorly motivated to seek diagnosis or treatment of venereal infection. They commonly are not dissuaded even by gross genital lesions from further sexual contact. They therefore constitute a high-prevalence group with great potential for disseminating venereal infection throughout the community. In institutions, they provide captive groups that are likely to give high yields on routine screening.

Attitudes and Beliefs

Although ignorance of sexual matters has been suggested as a contributing factor to promiscuity,[51] several studies have shown no relationship between knowledge of VD and infection.[52,53] One study even showed that infection was more common in those with a knowledge of VD.[54] Promiscuity and venereal infection are probably influenced far more by the attitudes of the individuals involved than by their knowledge.[7] These attitudes also influence readiness to seek treatment, reliability in taking medication, cooperation in contact tracing, and dissemination of infection before adequate treatment.[55,56] The attitudes of physicians and the general public, apart from their more general significance in venereal disease control, have an indirect influence through their effect on the patient. Shame, guilt, and consequent reluctance to acknowledge infection are still major features of the venereal diseases. This reticence hinders epidemiologic investigation, particularly where nonvaginal coitus is involved. The venereologist has little control over the intrinsic attitudes of the patient, but these attitudes should be fully considered when choosing therapy or in epidemiologic investigation. A dramatic favorable trend in patient attitudes can only be expected if medical and public attitudes moderate.

Promiscuity and venereal infection are often aggravated by irrational beliefs, Infection has been associated with the beliefs that satisfaction of sexual needs is essential to health and that the accumulation of semen is harmful.[37] The belief that masturbation is injurious may be more common in VD patients.[22] An inverse relationship between masturbation and infection has been noted.[57]

Beliefs tending to depress promiscuity are usually related to religion. Modern studies, however, have not shown a convincing relationship between venereal infection and either religious affiliation or depth of religious conviction. This probably relates to the limited impact of religious belief in modern society. Even in past times or among deeply religious individuals, religious conviction often has afforded little immunity from sexual desires or the sequelae of indulgence of such desires. Religion, therefore, has little influence on VD incidence, although in some individuals it magnifies the psychological problems associated with infection.[29]

Alcoholic Intake

"The association of drinking with casual promiscuity is revealed in the stories told by patients and contacts and by the behavior observed in houses which are most frequently named as meeting places."[58]

There is ample support to show a link between drinking and promiscuity. Reports commonly name hotels or bars as either the meeting place or site of intercourse for 20 percent–70 percent of VD patients.[59-62] Schofield[63] demonstrated a strong association (P less than 0.001) between sex activity and visiting a public bar. Of those with intercourse experience 75 percent had visited a bar in the past week whereas only 44 percent of those without intercourse experience had done so. However, a similar relationship between intercourse and cigarette smoking was also found. Twenty-seven percent of those with intercourse experience, compared with 58 percent of those without this experience, were nonsmokers. In spite of this association there is little reason to suspect a causal relationship between cigarette smoking and intercourse. This emphasizes the point that sexual activity and drinking are both dominant social activities in modern society. One might expect a strong association between them even in the absence of a causal relationship. This is not purely a chance association, however, as the aggregation of suitable clients makes bars and hotels ideal centers for prostitutes or those seeking casual liaisons. The sale of sex and sale of alcohol, since each enhances the other, are clearly symbiotic commercial practices.

The influence of alcohol on the susceptibility of the individual to casual unions or venereal infection is more controversial. Opinions vary from those who see the influence of alcohol as a prominent precipitant of venereal infection to those who consider drinking as merely an excuse used to explain behavior the individual or physician might otherwise consider unacceptable. Certainly the association between infection and alcohol is often impressive, *e.g.*, there was excessive alcoholic intake in 19 percent of VD patients compared to less than 1 percent of the controls.[31] Of patients, 29.5 percent were heavy drinkers and only 2 percent of the controls. Among VD patients 49 percent were intoxicated and 7 percent were totally drunk at the time of infection.[1]

The immediate influence of alcohol has other consequences besides actual exposure and infection. The experience among Australian troops in Vietnam demonstrates the diversity of this impact. Alcohol use was a serious problem in its own right, but in some ways, it may have alleviated the VD problem by providing an alternative leisure activity or form of social escapism. Sometimes it also rendered soldiers incapable of sexual participation. Its main influence on VD, however, was markedly adverse. It was probably a major influence on 50 percent of the soldiers having intercourse. Of those omitting prophylaxis, 25 percent did so because of drunkenness. Inebriation prevented 50 percent of VD sufferers from providing a useful contact report. Alcohol not only greatly increased the intercourse incidence but effectively thwarted any personal or community preventive campaign.

The studies cited above, however, have involved military personnel. Civilian experience is usually quite different. Soldiers, who are commonly heavy drinkers, often live in a disrupted environment in which periods of enforced abstinence are broken by brief intervals of over-indulgence—in both alcohol and sex. By contrast, civilians tend to be milder drinkers and to have a more uniform alcohol intake and sexual outlet. This difference is typified by the findings on venereal disease patients in New Guinea.[57] The soldiers mostly contracted their infections at places of entertainment at night or during weekends when they had been drinking. The civilians acquired infection from casual contacts at any time during the day; alcohol was rarely involved.

Apart from a direct association of alcohol, promiscuity, and VD, there is probably a relationship between patterns of drinking and promiscuity. This may be mediated by a third parameter such as personality. This hypothesis is supported by a close relationship between base-line alcohol intake (independent of intake at time of sexual contact) and intercourse with prostitutes.[29] Intercourse with prostitutes was experienced by approximately 50 percent of social drinkers and abstainers, by 72 percent of regular and heavy drinkers, and by 81 percent of very heavy drinkers.

It is clear, therefore, that the association of venereal disease and alcohol is complex, diverse, and variable from one community to another. In any community it is imperative to determine what contribution alcohol makes to the overall problem of control and to adjust any program accordingly. In some situations failure to consider the influence of alcohol may preclude effective control of venereal disease.

Personal Prophylaxis

For practical purposes, there are three categories of personal preventive measures: mechanical (of which the condom is the most important), local applications, and systemic chemotherapy.

In the sixteenth century Fallopio reported the first use of the condom to protect 1100 men from syphilis. Since this time the condom has been an important element of many control programs, particularly in wartime. Opposition to the condom has been expressed: "its effectiveness makes the condom useless as a prophylactic against gonorrhea, and even under ideal conditions against syphilis,"[64] but many would disagree with this view. Certainly condoms should be undamaged, of good quality, and used at the right time in the correct manner. Frequent failure of the condom to prevent VD can be attributed to deficiencies in these conditions.

The efficacy of the condom is suggested by several studies. Venereal infection was demonstrated in 9.5 percent of those using a condom or having early treatment, in 22 percent of those using inadequate prophylaxis, and in 68.5 percent of those using none.[1] A fall in the VD rate from 250 to 120 men, over a 4-month interval in one unit of 1200 men in Africa, was coincident with the distribution of 4000 sheaths. Among Australian troops in Vietnam, the incidence of condom usage in the general population (22.5 percent) was over five times greater than its use in various groups of VD patients (4 percent of clinic attenders, 4.5 percent of those completing trace reports, and 3.1 percent of a questionnaire series). In an interview study, the VD rate of those using a condom was nil compared to 30 percent for those utilizing local prophylaxis, and 26 percent for those using no prophylaxis.[52] Among teenagers in Denmark, condoms were used only one quarter as frequently by infected subjects as by controls.[36] In another study, T-mycoplasma were detected in 14.3 percent of condom users, but in 42.5 percent of those who did not use condoms.[65]

These findings are not inconsistent with the view that condoms probably have an insignificant effect on total venereal disease morbidity.[66] This low rate of effectiveness stems from the reluctance of many sexual participants to use this prophylaxis and from its incorrect use by many others.

In many environments condom use ranges from 3 percent–20 percent among VD clinic patients. It rarely exceeds 25 percent in the general male population.[67] Furthermore, condoms are used least by those who need them most. Juhlin[45] found that a condom was used by 44 percent of individuals who had one sex partner but by only 15 percent of those who were more promiscuous. Tables 8-1 and 8-2 show

TABLE 8-1 PROPHYLAXIS USAGE RELATED TO SEXUAL EXPOSURE
WITH VIETNAMESE PROSTITUTES[a]

Sexual exposures	Number	Percent Using			
		Condom always	Washing always	No prophylaxis	Prophylaxis Sometimes
1	65	38.5	21.5	40	0
2	37	24	16	54	0
3	38	24	5	34	37
4	16	12.5	12.5	19	56
5	17	18	—	29	53
6–10	49	10	10	33	47
11–20	14	7	—	64	29
Over 20	10	10	—	40	50

[a] Hart G: Factors influencing venereal infection in a war environment, Br J Vener Dis 50: 68, 1974

similar trends among both soldiers[52] and male college students.[65] Condom use progressively decreased from about 30 percent among those with few partners to about 7 percent among those with many partners.

In some countries condoms have very low acceptance among women[68] who may resort to breaking them before use,[26] but failure to use a condom is mainly related to the lack of initiative of the male. Table 8-3 summarizes the reasons for omission of prophylaxis in three studies. Impairment of pleasure was the main motivating factor in two other studies.[7,69] The embarrassment of obtaining a condom has also been suggested as a major deterrent.[34] Both beliefs and attitudes are largely responsible for prophylaxis omission. Among Australian troops

TABLE 8-2 CONDOM USAGE AMONG MALE COLLEGE STUDENTS[a]

Number of Sexual Partners	Number	Regular Condom Usage	
		Number	%
1	32	10	31
2	23	6	26
3–5	41	13	32
6–14	29	5	17
Over 14	15	1	7

[a] McCormack WM, Lee Y, Zinner SH: Sexual experience and urethral colonization with genital mycoplasmas, Ann Intern Med 78: 696, 1973

TABLE 8-3 REASONS FOR FAILURE TO USE A CONDOM[a]

Reason	Curjel[b]	Wittkower and Cowan[c]	Hart[d]
Not available	29	10	22
Considered infection unlikely	23	56	
Influence of alcohol	16	13	25
Impaired pleasure	13.5	17	35
Knew partner	6.5		
No fear of VD	5.5		
Ignorance	3.4		
Forgot			12.5

[a] Figures are given in percentages
[b] Curjel HE: An analysis of the human reasons underlying the failure to use a condom in 723 cases of venereal disease, J R Nav Med Serv 50: 203, 1964
[c] Wittkower ED, Cowan J: Some psychological aspects of sexual promiscuity, Psychosom Med 6: 287, 1944
[d] Hart G: Factors influencing venereal infection in a war environment, Br J Vener Dis 50: 68, 1974

in Vietnam only 30 percent of both clinic patients and controls considered the condom to be highly effective. More important, only 22 percent of those with faith in condoms actually used them.

The strong inverse relationship between condom usage and venereal infection may not be a causal one. They both relate to attitudes and other behavioral determinants. At present these are poorly understood and have so far proven resistant to therapeutic manipulation.

Local prophylactic procedures involve urination plus liberal applications of soap and water to the genitalia and adjacent areas, or the application of permanganate or salts of silver or mercury to the urethra and external genitalia. Prior to the antibiotic era, both therapy and prevention depended solely on these methods, and there have been impressive claims for their effectiveness.

Crede first used installation of silver nitrate to prevent gonococcal ophthalmia neonatorum in 1882; this has been used effectively ever since. Prior to antibiotics, silver nitrate was widely used for both prevention and treatment of gonococcal genital infections. In 1904, Metchnikoff and Roux established the value of 33 percent calomel solution as a prophylactic against syphilis.

These chemical prophylactics were usually administered from prophylactic centers, which were situated in the soldiers' lines or near sites of exposure. The centers were identified by signs or colored lighting, were open continuously, and were sometimes manned by an attendant. Soldiers also carried personal prophylactic kits. Commonly used preparations in the prophylactic stations were 2 percent silver protein, 1:4000 potassium permanganate, and 33 percent calomel cream. Douches of permanganate were sometimes used by females. Prophylactic kits utilized 0.25 percent silver nitrate jelly, or calomel ointment, and Argyrol.

It might be expected that the efficacy of these methods would depend largely on the thoroughness with which they were instituted and the time lag following intercourse. Dunham[70] suggested that application should occur within one hour of exposure but that some benefit could be expected if application occurred within 5–6 hours.

Claims for the effectiveness of these measures include a reduction of the VD rate in World War I from 625/1000 by the compulsory application of prophylaxis to all men returning from leave, regardless of exposure. There was an infection rate of 1 in 37 exposures without prophylaxis but 1 in 274 exposures with prophylaxis.[71] Among Australian troops in Syria in World War II, for nearly 8 weeks more than 400 soldiers used ablution centers daily. A total of 18,000 treatments were given. Only 61 of these patients contracted VD.[72] In a controlled brothel in World War II, venereal disease was acquired by only 87 of 248,593 troops using the ablutive center (0.31/1000 exposures). The estimated VD rate for those not using ablution was 0.72/1000 exposures.[73] Among British troops in Southeast Asia a high VD rate followed when reduced utilization of prophylactic packets took place.[11] Very few British soldiers in the Middle East in World War II contracted syphilis or gonorrhea when they used a treatment center within 2 hours of coitus.[74]

There are limitations on the effectiveness of local applications. Wittkower and Cowan[1] consider washing genitalia and flushing the urethra inadequate. Patients using these methods had an infection rate of 22 percent compared with 9.5 percent for those using a condom. Willcox[26] suggested prophylactic centers were a failure. In one unit, 40 percent had gonorrhea by the time they used the facilities and they attended only to avoid disciplinary action. In another unit, every man had compulsory prophylaxis regardless of whether he had intercourse. In spite of this, there was no reduction in the VD rate in 3 months. Prophylactic kits were phased out of the U.S. Army in 1959,[9] presumably because of their lack of effectiveness. Washing was of little use as utilized by Australian troops in Vietnam.[52] In several studies those using washing as prophylaxis had VD rates similar to those who did not.

Among American soldiers in Italy, the main objections to attending prophylactic stations were 1) the belief that condom usage was sufficient, 2) the embarrassment of queueing in public, 3) objection to sanitary conditions at the station, 4) the harmful effect of chemicals on genitals, and 5) the fear of consequences of disclosure of attendance.[7] These reasons are more rational than those usually volunteered for omission of condom prophylaxis. Due to the obvious shortcomings of presently available methods, local applications should be discarded. At best they provide a false sense of security, and they may result in actual harm to the patient. Even if a totally effective, nontoxic application were available, it is doubtful if it would make a significant contribution to venereal disease control for it would suffer the same shortcomings of utilization as the condom.

There can be little doubt that systemic chemotherapy is the most effective form of prophylaxis,[75,76] and that smaller doses are effective for this purpose than are required for the cure of an established infection.[78] These advantages are offset by some very significant defects. A large distribution of expensive antibiotics may be involved. Since these will be used for all exposures, the total amount used may greatly exceed the amount required if only established infections are treated. The possibility exists that improper usage may facilitate the emergence of resistant strains. The clinical picture may be confused, complicating adequate management. Associated with the above factors, there may be a great increase in venereoneurosis among those exposed to infection.

The role of preventive methods in controlling venereal disease is uncertain.[67] The impact of effective prophylactics on disease incidence depends more on which particular individuals use them than on the proportion of the total population who do so. The low use of effective prophylactics, particularly by promiscuous individuals, has restricted their influence on disease control in the past. Since universal utilization is unlikely, their potential impact is complex and difficult to predict.

Chapter Nine

Psychological
Aspects
of
Venereal Disease

Psychological factors are important in determining the types of individuals which are particularly susceptible to infection. These factors also influence the response of individuals after venereal exposure.

An abnormal incidence of psychiatric parameters has been noted in VD patients—in one study 43 percent of patients, compared to 5 percent of controls, had been previously referred to a psychiatrist.[1] Most attention, however, has focused on the relationship between personality and risk of infection.

Personality

The suspected association between personality and infection, particularly recurrent infection, is revealed in many writings:

"Officers with V.D. were almost invariably either socially maladjusted or inadequate personalities with poor service records."

"Almost all the cases of repeated infection occurred amongst the psychopaths, aggressives or socially maladjusted groups."[2]

"It's the odds and sods who get it."[3]

"A good soldier may get V.D. However, if a man gets V.D. twice or more often, it indicates a weak personality because he does not learn by experience."[1]

141

Venereal infection is certainly related directly to the sociopathic personality—the underlying disorder in habitual promiscuity (Chapter 5). Quite predictably, of soldiers discharged from the Canadian Army with a diagnosis of psychopathic personality, 25 percent had had venereal disease. Of those discharged with neurosis, only 3 percent had been infected.[1]

Eysenck's[4,5] refinement of the personality inventory has provided a useful tool for measuring certain personality components— extraversion, neuroticism, and psychoticism. According to Eysenck's[6] theories, "extraversion constitutes a major dimension of personality related to criminal and generally anti-social behaviour." Some specific hypotheses arise from these theories: extraverts will have intercourse earlier than introverts; extraverts will have intercourse more frequently than introverts; extraverts will have intercourse with a greater number of different persons per unit time; extraverts will have intercourse in more diverse positions than introverts; and extraverts will indulge in more varied sexual behavior outside intercourse (so-called perversions).[6]

With respect to neuroticism, these predictions are that "high N [neurotic] scorers are characterized by a labile autonomic system, and are thus susceptible to fear and anxiety to a degree which may make them less likely to indulge in sexual behaviour, particularly outside the legal bounds of matrimony."[6] Several independent studies have confirmed that inventory findings are related in a consistent pattern to a wide variety of sexual behavior and its sequelae.[7-12]

Extraversion is a prominent feature of behavior associated with the VD patient. Extraverts begin intercourse at an early age, practice fellatio and cunnilingus frequently, masturbate infrequently, and are likely to acquire venereal infection in both stable and stressful environments. Predictably, soldiers tend to score more highly for extraversion than civilians. Introversion is a specific feature of those reluctant to engage in overt sexuality. Introverts often first experience intercourse in their twenties and tend to avoid promiscuous heterosexual behavior even in stressful situations. Introversion is common in homosexuals.

Neuroticism is also associated with venereal infection but is a more prominent feature of those who engage in practices of limited social acceptability and who exhibit neurotic manifestations after venereal exposure. Neuroticism is associated with excess masturbation, passive homosexuality, and intimate sexual behavior in public. Excessive guilt, shame, worry, refusal to accept reassurance and obsessive acts after exposure are features of neurotic individuals. In summary, individuals whose personality scores fall in the high extraversion–high neuroticism quadrant contribute disproportionately to the morbidity from venereal exposure (Figure 9-1).

Similar trends in personality occur both with other forms of behavior that are often considered deviant and with parameters which have previously been associated with venereal disease patients. Figure 9-2 demonstrates graphically this similarity in trends for venereal disease, alcohol intake, education, age, and military and civil offences. Increased extraversion is associated with venereal infection, greater alcoholic intake, lower education, lower age, larger numbers of military and civil offences. There is a general tendency for similar trends in neuroticism, although this tendency is not marked for all parameters.

These findings suggest that the relationship of certain sociological parameters to venereal infection may be of a secondary nature, in so far as all are related primarily to the personality of the individual. The precise relationship between clinical categories of personality and inventory findings is not critical to this argument. Without defining the actual personality, it is possible to say that certain personality types, which can be represented by particular inventory scores, are prone to certain behavior usually regarded as antisocial, viz., venereal disease, civil arrests, frequent military charges, and excessive alcohol intake. Further studies may produce similar findings for other behavior patterns, e.g., drug dependence, delinquency, and criminal behavior.

This further highlights the need to consider venereal disease as a behavioral problem, the control of which requires focus on the fundamental personality of the individual. Attempts to alter other parameters that also depend on personality may be inappropriate and meet with failure.

Psychosocial Reactions to Venereal Exposure

Clinicians frequently overlook the psychological sequelae of exposure to venereal infection and consequently adopt a therapeutic approach quite inappropriate to the needs of their patients. This oversight may reinforce any existing neuroses and make subsequent cure more difficult. Psychological reaction to venereal infection is very common. It occurs in up to 85 percent of patients[13-15] and often outweighs any physical disability. In some environments neurotic manifestations are even more severe in promiscuous individuals who do not acquire VD.[16] Consequently, psychological sequelae to venereal exposure, although poorly understood, frequently unrecognized, and inadequately managed, are among the most common conditions encountered in medical practice. These common sequelae should not be

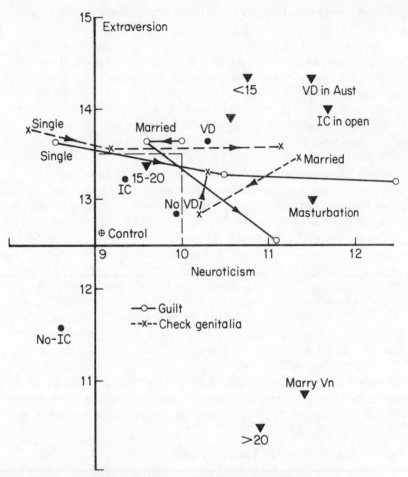

FIGURE 9–1 EXTRAVERSION—NEUROTICISM TRENDS FOR VARIOUS GROUPS

(i) ● Subgroups of control series (i.c. and no-i.c.) and of clinic series (VD and No-VD), ⊕ Overall mean of control group. (ii) ▼ Divisions within the clinic series: (a) Age of first intercourse (<15, 15–20, >20); (b) Venereal infection in Australia; (c) Those practicing fellatio; (d) Frequent masturbators; (e) Those keen to marry Vietnamese; (f) Those having intercourse in the open. (iii) –○–Degrees of guilt of married and single soldiers. The arrows indicating increasing guilt following intercourse, from never to sometimes to often. ...X...Degrees of checking genitalia of married and single soldiers. The arrows indicating increasing checking of genitalia following intercourse, from never, to a little, to a lot.

From Soc. Sci. Med., 1973, Vol. 7, p.458; reproduced with permission of the Editor.

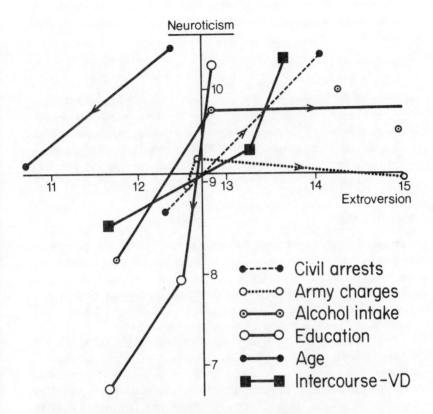

FIGURE 9-2 TRENDS OF EXTRAVERSION AND NEUROTICISM
Varying involvement in the prostitution-venereal disease environment is compared with those for civil arrests, military charges, alcohol intake, education, and age.

From Brit. J. Vener. Dis., Vol. 49, p. 552, 1973; reproduced with permission of the Editor.

confused with preexisting psychiatric disturbances of VD patients, which are relatively uncommon and differ in both etiology and management.

Some patients show only mild concern which responds readily to reassurance. This is the same response as that presented by patients with most other diseases when there may be initial concern over prognosis if the disability is encountered for the first time. The frequency of this response varies markedly from one environment to another. In some settings it may occur in only a minority of exposed individuals.

Other responses to venereal infection may be considered abnormal.

Since these sequelae are both diverse and complex, it is helpful to subdivide them into three groups—no reaction, underreaction, and overreaction.

No Reaction

Repeated venereal infection may represent a relatively insignificant facet of the incorrigible sociopath who is a social hazard because of his more general behavioral maladjustment. These individuals are habitually promiscuous—discarding each casual partner immediately after intercourse and moving to another. Their sexual behavior resembles masturbatory gratification, and their promiscuity represents a search for the unobtainable.[17] This problem has been discussed more fully in Chapter 5.

Underreaction

Underreaction to venereal infection is manifest as apathy or bravado.[2] Apathy is the most frequent reaction in underdeveloped countries or in underprivileged communities. It has been reported from New Guinea[18] and India.[19] These patients disregard therapy for months and continue to have intercourse despite gross genital lesions. Bravado was a frequent reaction in military circles, and membership in a Swedish military officers club depended on proof of previous syphilitic infection.[20] In some societies venereal infection is considered a prerequisite for manhood.[21]

Delay in seeking treatment often has very serious consequences for the individual. In New Guinea, patients with Donovanosis often delay seeking treatment for months. In India, 73 percent of patients with this condition waited for more than 2 months before attending a VD clinic.[22] The gross permanent structural sequelae of this condition, including complete erosion of the genitalia and urethral occlusion, are attributable solely to delay in seeking treatment.

However, attitudes to venereal infection have public health implications as well as personal consequences. Apathy may account for the reduced reported incidence of nongonococcal urethritis (NGU) in some ethnic groups. The milder symptoms and the spontaneous remission rate may cause the patient to disregard symptoms and seek no treatment. In New Guinea, NGU was rarely seen in civilian patients attending a venereal disease clinic.[18] A study of Reiter's disease frequently disclosed NGU on examination, although the patients had not previously complained of the condition.[23] In soldiers, who had greater access to medical care and who were subjected to routine physical examinations, NGU was common. A similar mechanism may account for the rarity with which this condition is reported from the Navajo Indian population[24] and for its decreased contribution to urethritis in the black as compared to the white American population.[25]

Since the syphilis chancre is usually painless and heals spontaneously in a few weeks, apathetic patients with this condition probably will be reluctant to seek treatment. In some communities a higher proportion of syphilis is detected by physical examination or screening in the later (secondary or latent) stages. In New Guinea, primary syphilis was rarely seen, but routine examination and serologic screening of prostitutes and soldiers demonstrated significant prevalence of syphilis in the population. In fiscal year 1974 (FY74), the ratio of primary syphilis to early latent syphilis was only 0.81 among Navajo[24] men compared with 1.98 among white American men.[26]

Delay in seeking treatment for gonococcal infection probably increases the incidence of complications. Since the introduction of antibiotics, the changing sex distribution of disseminated infection from predominantly men to predominantly women has been attributed to the reduced duration of infection in men, who now seek early treatment of acute urethritis.[27] Although recent studies of gonococcal arthritis have shown a predominance of women (79 percent in one study[27]), approximately equal numbers of men and women among the Navajo (48 percent were men in FY74)[24] are hospitalized for this condition. This suggests that the delay in treatment caused by the asymptomatic nature of infection in the women may be balanced by the men's failure to respond to symptoms.

Overreaction

Psychopathology. Overreaction is the most common sequel to exposure. These patients can be divided into those who are more concerned over their behavioral lapse (the morally oriented) and those who react to venereal infection (VD oriented).

Often the morally oriented patients have experienced an isolated casual sexual contact and are disturbed at their own "tarnished" self-image. They may actually desire venereal infection as a sadomasochistic solution to their guilt.[28] Menninger[29] cites cases of a college student with gonorrhea interrupting treatment to avoid being cured too quickly, and another who behaved "as if he wanted to hang onto his infection." Guilt may be experienced more by those who do not acquire VD, which is seen by some as a form of expiation. Venereal infection may be a relief; the crisis may be faced openly, and the cure of infection heralds the conclusion of the episode. Those escaping infection continue to worry, check their genitalia, experience shame, and do not know the duration of their penance.

Patients orientated toward venereal disease are primarily concerned with escaping infection and its sequelae. This concern is manifested as fear, shame, or aggression. In the fear reaction, the patient fears damage to himself (sterility, impotence, irrevocable contamination)[30] or to his associates (lover, wife, children). Belief in the sin or disgrace of VD produces shame and fear of discovery by friends or family. This guilt may arise from intercourse on a casual basis or it may be associated with particular sexual practices (masturbation, sodomy, or orogenital acts). In general, VD patients tend to be more aggressive than others,[31] but some tend to blame the world and society for all their problems.[32] They are grandiose, demanding, rebellious, uncooperative, and self-pitying. They may show marked hostility to medical attendants and toward the partner who transmitted their infection. Revenge may be demonstrated by refusal to disclose the contact so that others will be exposed to infection, homicidal assault on the partner, and the deliberate exposure of uninfected partners.

Clinical syndromes.

Overreaction to venereal exposure may manifest itself as venereoneurosis or as more severe disturbance.

Venereoneurosis. Persons with a venereoneurotic reaction are those who having been exposed to venereal infection are preoccupied with bodily processes which they imagine indicate the onset of incomplete cure of venereal disease. In addition, these persons may perform persistent irrational acts designed to confirm or negate their fears.[11] Irrational concern is focused on symptoms attributed to urethral discharge or the appearance and sensations of the genitalia.[33] Anxiety and hypochondriasis are common features, and there is usually an obsessive-compulsive element to these manifestations.

The components involved in venereoneurosis include urethrorrhea, penile manipulation, penile structures, and demand for treatment. Any urethral discharge, even a minute quantity of clear serous fluid, appearing at any time after intercourse may be considered a grave omen by the anxious patient. This often appears in association with defecation but may be noticed at other times. Patients commonly mention a drop of clear discharge protruding from the urinary meatus or adherent lips of the meatus on waking each morning. Frequently intermittent urethral discharge follows effective treatment of infectious urethritis. Classically, this discharge is clear or milky, occurs in small quantities at infrequent intervals, and is unaccompanied by other symptoms. Acceptance of these symptoms (or the patient's description of these symptoms) as indicative of persistent venereal disease without objective evidence of relapse and subsequent administration of further antibiotic therapy may lead to an extended process of diverse drug therapy and to considerable emotion on the part of the patient. Such a situation usually terminates with both doctor and patient dissatisfied. Penile massage or swabs inserted into the urethra to obtain culture samples may be sufficient to maintain a small amount of discharge and confirm the patient's fears that his venereal infection has not been cured. If this situation prevails for some time, it becomes difficult to convince the patient that his preoccupation and anxiety are responsible for the perpetuation of spurious indicators of nonexistent disease.

Physicians will continue to aggravate neurotic tendencies in patients unless they are aware of these manifestations. They must apply precise diagnostic and treatment criteria for the venereal diseases, in particular nongonococcal urethritis. The diagnosis of nongonococcal urethritis should not be made in the absence of objective criteria, *e.g.,* isolation of a causative organism or numerous polymorphs in a Gram-stained smear. The significance of occasional polymorphs in a urethral smear from a patient who is asymptomatic or has minimal urethral discharge must be evaluated against the background of the patient's recent experiences (sexual exposure, penile manipulation, intraurethral chemicals or swabs). They do not necessarily indicate antibiotic therapy.

Penile manipulation is important both as a marker of venereo-neurosis and as a direct contributor to the production of urethral discharge. Most commonly the penis is not milked from base to meatus but merely squeezed vigorously around the glans or distal end of the shaft. This may be performed when showering, before urination, when in bed or, in more severe cases of anxiety, routinely throughout the day. When performed by patients recovering from urethritis this added mechanical irritation is usually sufficient to produce some exudate at the meatus and confirm the patient's fears of persisting VD. Proponents of this practice usually identify themselves when asked to produce some discharge from the penis. In contrast to the cautious manipulation of other patients, these individuals attack the organ with such vigor, squeezing the glans or wringing the whole shaft, that they appear intent on its destruction.

Some individuals present with penile pain as a result of close analysis of their sensations. Others present because of penile conditions that have been located by equally thorough visual scrutiny. The slightest irregularity in pigmentation or skin surface is often considered of awesome significance. Skin tags, hair follicles, and sebaceous cysts commonly cause concern, and the existence of pearly penile papules on the glans often prompt the request for treatment of penile warts. Some patients are so distressed or convinced that they have been infected that they request, or commonly demand treatment. When there is no indication for treatment, such a demand is a fairly ominous manifestation of venereoneurosis, since these individuals tend to be more severely disturbed and have a worse prognosis than some other neurotics.

Severe depressive conditions. Frank psychiatric syndromes,[34] hospitalization, and suicide[35-37] sometimes occur as sequelae to venereal exposure. Depression, melancholia, and phobia may occur, but the cardinal feature is the patient's strong conviction that he is venereally infected.

Pedder[38] has suggested that the most likely psychiatric explanation in these cases is that the patients had preexisting severe depressive conditions. The fear of venereal disease is merely a part of this illness rather than its cause. This is certainly true in some cases, but it appears unlikely in others. The two groups can usually be distinguished if a precise history is available. The psychotic individual who has a past history of hypochondriasis or develops fears of other diseases besides VD clearly belongs in the former group. When the onset of symptoms in a previously sound individual can be traced to a definite sexual episode, a direct etiologic relationship is more likely. This situation arises most commonly when an individual acts in an atypical manner during a period of stress, *e.g.,* visiting a prostitute during a period of prolonged absence from wife or steady sex partner.[39]

Management

Overreaction to venereal exposure is largely iatrogenic, for inadequate management will foster neurosis in the normal patient and will aggravate preexisting neurosis. A neurotic patient often reflects the uncertainty, indecision, and ignorance of the medical attendant. All patients require investigation of their psychological, as well as their physical problem; however, venereoneurosis has its origins, and is most amenable to treatment, in the period immediately after exposure. The management of venereoneurosis requires a thorough knowledge of the natural course and treatment of venereal disease, and consequently, the condition should be managed by the venereologist. Delegation of this responsibility to the psychiatrist complicates rather than solves the problem.

The first interview is the most critical period of management, and the development of a positive doctor–patient relationship is the most vital component of this interview.[40] If the patient feels he is unable to relate to his attendant, there is little chance that he will be managed adequately.

A thorough history and examination of the patient are essential. These provide an accurate diagnosis, but more importantly they allow ventilation of his concerns by the patient. This has therapeutic value, and it directs the clinician's attention to areas of psychological trouble. It is essential for the physician to listen to all of the patient's complaints and worries, and the patient must be encouraged to verbalize any anxieties.

Prophylactic reassurance at a low level, and prediction in general terms of the course of the illness are helpful. It is important to mention physiological or benign conditions that may be mistaken for venereal disease and to discuss any intermittent transient symptoms which may sometimes occur following the successful treatment of infection. Patients should be routinely instructed as to the possible exacerbation of symptoms by frequently squeezing the penis, excess alcohol, and vigorous exercise in the initial stages of their infection. They should be reassured that a thorough assessment of their progress will be made at their surveillance visits and that they should not be unduly concerned in the interim. This routine is time-consuming but markedly reduces the incidence of venereoneurosis.[11]

The established psychoneurotic requires treatment for his psychiatric condition and not for his imagined physical illness. Placebos, antibiotics, and multiple pathology investigations are therefore contraindicated, since they undermine psychotherapy and reinforce belief in the physical nature of the illness. Similarly, therapeutic reassurance is harmful because it may produce a credibility gap and damage the doctor–patient relationship.[41] Of course the neurotic patient is not immune from future infection, and further exposure or the development of objective signs should be investigated in the normal manner.

The patient who has a longstanding conviction that he is chronically infected with venereal disease is in special danger. If he does not have a positive relationship with his physician, and particularly if he continues to move from one physician to another, he poses a definite suicide risk. In contrast to the venereoneurotic, these individuals should be referred for psychiatric management as soon as their condition is recognized. Regardless of management, the prognosis is poor.

Public education programs have the potential for both alleviating and aggravating the psychological sequelae of venereal exposure. The type of propaganda that is likely to foster some concern and so be beneficial for the apathetic patient is unlikely to console the venereoneurotic. Nonselective publicity campaigns which stress fear or undue concern about VD may create more problems than they solve. Attendance at VD clinics may increase by up to 100 percent, but most of the additional patients do not have VD.[42] This increased work load to process uninfected individuals diverts staff from more rewarding activities. Much time may be required also to reassure these same individuals in whom undue concern has been fostered.

Chapter Ten

Special Groups

In most communities there are special high-risk groups whose members contribute disproportionately to the venereal disease incidence. The identification of these groups and appropriate measures to reduce the incidence of venereal disease within them are essential components of any control program. There are a few very large groups which by their very nature tend to be involved with venereal disease. It is important to have an understanding of the sociological dynamics responsible for this association.

Teenagers

"The primary dilemma for young people is that they have great individual freedom but are not supposed to have coitus."[1]

Teenagers are frequently blamed as a dominant group in the resurgence of venereal disease in recent years. Impressive statistics have been quoted, *e.g.*, in 1961, the 15–19 year age group contributed 43 percent of the female gonorrhea in Denmark and 26 percent of the female gonorrhea in England and Wales.[2] These data superficially appear to support the charge against teenagers. There are so many variables with a direct influence on these figures that they are worthless as indicators of promiscuity or its sequelae within any group. For instance, it may well be that these figures reflect a greater detection or reporting of venereal disease within the teenage group. This age group may form a high proportion of the sexually active members of the community. They may perform a high proportion of the sexual acts within the community. Certainly by removing some of these variables, a more realistic appreciation of the teenage contribution may be obtained. A fairly consistent pattern found in many countries is a peak rate in the 20–24 age group with moderately high rates among teenagers and lower rates among older groups. This pattern is typified by the 1971 syphilis rates in the United States and the gonorrhea rates in Canada—the respective rates per 100,000 among teenagers were 19.8 and 20.4 compared with 41.3 and 36.9 in the 20–24 age group.[3]

Possibly the focus on teenagers has resulted from a marked increase in venereal disease among this group. Table 10-1 shows that while this is so, the relative increase is less than that in both the 20–24 age group and in the general population. The special attention given to teenagers must therefore have. its origins in factors other than the infection rate. Certainly the number of teenagers has increased, a greater proportion are indulging in sexual relations, and they are more open

TABLE 10–1   REPORTED INCIDENCE OF VENEREAL DISEASE IN THE
UNITED STATES (Case Rates per 100,000)[a]

Age Group	Primary and Secondary Syphilis			Gonorrhea		
	1956	1968	% increase	1956	1968	% increase
15–19 years	10.7	19.3	80	415.7	610.6	47
20–24 years	18.4	38.8	111	781.8	1251.1	60
over 24 years	3.6	9.4	161	106.9	165.6	55
Total	3.9	9.6	146	135.7	235.1	74

[a] Quoted in Willcox RR: A world look at the venereal diseases, Med Clin North Am 5: 1057, 1972

about sexual behavior and its sequelae than older groups. Public awareness of teenage sexuality and venereal disease is consequently greater than ever before. The real reason for concern over teenage venereal disease, however, becomes apparent when the suggested reasons for this phenomenon are considered.[2] These reasons have been given as ignorance of sex and abuse of the sexual function, decline in religious faith, emancipation of the female, lack of discipline in home life and of parental supervision, the failure of fear as a deterrent, an emphasis on sexuality in books, films, and advertisements, and misinterpretation of psychological teaching, leading to the belief that self-restraint damages the personality. While these factors have undoubtedly contributed, it is noteworthy that they have a strong moralistic bias in common. More importantly, these same convictions, which were highly effective in modifying teenage behavior in the past, no longer have any influence. The key factor, therefore, is the revolutionary change in teenage attitudes. This change is apparent in all social groups in many different societies. The ethical and moral premises previously accepted as unchallengeable have now been challenged. The older generation cannot understand these new attitudes and refuses to accept them.

Among modern teenagers, sex with affection has widespread acceptance. The types of relationship that once permitted kissing only as acceptable behavior, later permitted petting and now permit vaginal and extravaginal coitus. Many individuals even use sex as a form of social expression in the absence of an affectionate relationship. To a few teenagers this behavior is not only acceptable but is considered as their right. A week or two of abstinence suggested by the venereologist is viewed as a considerable hardship.

As in other situations, idleness contributes to promiscuity and venereal disease. Many of the teenagers seen in clinics have few, if any absorbing interests. Their spare time often represents a period of boredom from which sexual indulgence provides the only relief. Some have a reluctance to seek or maintain employment and are content to live on welfare benefits or the benevolence of their parents and friends. With this limited social contact, they are strongly dependent on acceptance and encouragement from a circumscribed peer group whose members have attitudes and standards similar to their own. There are usually strong pressures within these groups to indulge in a variety of sexual behavior. There is a surprising ignorance, even among the more intelligent teenagers, of the potential hazards of this behavior and the methods by which they may be minimized.

The key factor in the management of the venereal disease problem among teenagers is their antiauthoritarian attitude. Their whole attitudinal and behavioral pattern represents a revolt against parental and societal values and the attempted implementation of these. If the epidemiologist adopts an authoritarian approach, he firmly identifies himself as an antagonist and is unlikely to receive significant cooperation from his teenage clients. Certainly criticism of the patient's attitudes or behavior and their suggested modification will serve no useful purpose. Regardless of his own personal beliefs, the physician must accept the attitudes and behavior of the teenager and offer his services in alleviating the problems of maladjustment which arise. The passive approach usually has a remarkable effect on the patient and does much to melt the facade of competence and sophistication that precludes assessment of the real problems confronting the individual. It is then possible to make some long-term impact on the behavioral patterns responsible for the high rate of venereal infection.

Immigrants

> "It is indeed well known that special temptations assail those who are temporarily or permanently separated from their families and homes."[4]

The contribution of migrants to venereal disease incidence is typified by the experience in Great Britain where, among males in 1968, 42 percent of gonococcal infections and 35 percent of infectious syphilis occurred in immigrant groups, of whom West Indians were the most numerous.[5] Imported infection makes only a minor contribution to this phenomenon, which depends mostly on the social stress confronting the new arrival in any country. Promiscuity and venereal disease have been attributed to the reduced inhibitions from parental, marital, tribal, religious, and other influences, but of course the main reason is removal of the sexual partner. The new arrival, particularly if he belongs to a distinctive racial group, is often treated as somewhat of an outcast. He rarely has access to the respectable females of his new country for social, much less sexual, purposes. Consequently he must rely on prostitutes or casual contacts with promiscuous females. In either case, there is a high risk of contracting venereal infection. If promiscuous females are not available, sexual outlet is dependent on homosexual behavior within the immigrant group.

A similar phenomenon has been noted in developing countries.[6,7] Large numbers of males, unaccompanied by their wives, are moved from rural areas to meet the labor demands of urban development. Although still in their own country, these laborers often experience a degree of social isolation greater than that experienced by the average migrant. Rigid tribal barriers deter harmonious social relationships even with the local males. Intimate contact with the females of the urban community is virtually precluded. The impact of this situation has been classically demonstrated in Port Moresby, the first city of Papua New Guinea. The influx of unaccompanied rural laborers resulted in a 62 percent excess male population in the community by 1972. Homosexual behavior was very common in these workers, and it made a significant contribution to the prevalence of Donovanosis, probably as common in this region as anywhere else in the world. With the obvious commercial potential in this unbalanced population, prostitution developed in the local populace. More recently, a few rural women have been imported. Although this has favored greater heterosexual outlet, it has had little impact on venereal disease except possibly to produce a little more gonorrhea and syphilis at the expense of Donovanosis. In this city almost the whole problem of venereal disease can be attributed to a social situation arising directly from rapid urban development and consequent unbalanced migration. In 1972, 93.5 percent of infections in male civilians and 100 percent in military patients occurred in those coming from rural areas.

Clearly the solution to this problem is to restore or maintain an even sex distribution in the community by insisting that immigrants bring their wives or sexual partners with them when they move to a new community. Where this tactic has been implemented, the increasing contribution of the migrant sector to venereal disease incidence has been arrested or the trend reversed.

Venereal disease is not the only adverse manifestation of unbalanced migration. All forms of crime, physical and mental illness, and general discontent are fostered by this situation. The total cost to the community of these sequelae far exceeds the initial outlay required to transport and accommodate the families of the migrating laborers.

This situation may be alleviated alternatively by a greater acceptance of immigrants into their new community. It is of doubtful benefit to a community to import individuals whom they are not prepared to accept socially. The initial economic or political gains from immigration will soon be outweighed by the disastrous social consequences inevitably associated with interracial or intertribal antagonism.

The Military

"Venereal disease among military personnel has been a serious problem from the era of the Greek city states to the present time."[8]

The military are clearly the most important single group involved with venereal disease. The incidence of military infection dwarfs that encountered in civilians. Where a civilian incidence of 50/100,000 in the sexually most active 20–24 age group is considered high, an infection rate 100 times this level is considered mild by military standards. The average army doctor may see more cases of VD than the venereologist in the same period. In one year he is likely to see more cases than the average civilian doctor sees in a lifetime. Despite centuries of association with VD, an almost paranoid obsession with incidence, and an outlay of enormous expenditure and manpower, military organizations have made an insignificant impact on the problem. For these reasons it is appropriate to consider in some detail the factors responsible for this persistent high incidence. There are three major aspects of this phenomenon.

Environmental stress. The environmental stress to which the soldier is often subjected has been fully discussed in Chapter 8. As mentioned there, controlled comparison demonstrates that this stress is directly responsible for a high proportion of venereal infection, particularly in wartime.

The soldier. Even in peacetime, venereal disease is more common in soldiers than in civilians. The general impression of those associated with soldiers is that they are considerably different from their civilian counterparts. It has often been suggested that their differences in behavior and its after-effects, including venereal infection, were largely due to these individual differences. A more precise demonstration of this view is offered by a comparison of Australian volunteers and conscripts in Vietnam where both groups were subjected to an identical environmental situation. While the social details of these findings are likely to vary in different communities, their general implications are probably applicable to the soldiers of most countries.

> The professional soldier is prone to venereal disease because of his characteristic sociological background—from a large family, limited education and indulgence in intercourse at an early age. His behavior is not markedly restricted by parental disapproval or marriage vows; he is reluctant to use masturbation as the major sexual outlet and shows little discrimination in acquiring sexual partners. He contributes disproportionately to the venereal disease problem both in his stable homeland environment and when he goes to war.[9]

Military policy and attitudes. Military society has always been characterized by certain distinctive qualities. Aggression and arrogance are viewed favorably; policy is implemented by power and punishment; moderation, compassion, tolerance, and understanding are viewed as weaknesses. The abysmal failure of the military in curbing venereal disease, alcoholism, drug addiction, or any other behavioral disorder is directly attributable to these attitudes, which may have won wars but are not conducive to the solution of social problems. The policies arising from these attitudes persist today, although their actual form has gradually changed.

The keystone of military policy is the view that venereal infection is a crime for which either the soldier or his responsible superior must be punished. Traditionally this punishment took the form of detention, fines, and loss of leave. The eighteenth-century French officer lost five-sixths of his salary and noncommissioned officers forfeited all their pay while hospitalized. Those with repeated infections were forced to extend their army service by a number of months equivalent to the days their infection had required treatment.[10] In the twentieth century, American soldiers with VD were court martialed. Venereal disease in his unit was accepted as a direct reflection on the military commander. Although Congress repealed the act for the punishment of individuals with venereal disease in 1944, reference to the efficiency of the commanding officer persisted for a further 10 years. British and Australian measures in this century have included imprisonment, stoppage of pay, and withdrawal of leave. Gradual reduction of these gross penalties has been achieved against the persistent opposition of combat officers.

More subtle pressures have been used and are currently achieving greater importance because of the abolition of the harsher penalties. In the Cuban headquarters in 1900, American troops were submitted to a weekly physical inspection, and the names of those with venereal disease posted on a bulletin board.[11] Among Australian troops in Vietnam, combat officers waged a persistent battle to obtain the names of their soldiers who had acquired infection. They almost achieved this aim on several occasions. In the absence of this information, some officers refused to cooperate in efforts to control venereal infection. It was envisaged that this information would enable moralistic counseling by the commanding officer, the elimination of some soldiers as candidates for key positions, and "appropriate" action against officers who became infected. For those with multiple infections, psychiatric referral and removal from the war theater have been advocated.

The result of all these policies is concealment of disease, illicit treatment, or self-treatment. The policies persist, therefore, because the military mind sees unequivocal proof of the success of punitive action: the harsher the penalties, the greater the reduction in reported incidence. As Greenberg[11] summarizes, "Consequently, the pressures that were applied in many instances drove venereal disease underground and resulted in eminently respectable, if totally misleading, rates."

While military authorities have concentrated on punishment for those who have become infected, fear has been utilized as the major deterrent. The regular VD film or lecture given by a combat officer, padre, or medical officer has become firmly entrenched in military campaigns against venereal disease. The lecturer is usually exhorted to emphasize the incurable strain and the ghastly sequelae resulting from an infection that may have initially been asymptomatic. It is unfortunate that most army officers still have great faith in this approach, even though expert opposition has been voiced for decades.

In 1909, Havard[12] wrote, "It is notorious that the influence of fear is a deterrent factor of slight importance." Wittkower and Cowan[13] have summarized the shortcoming of both fear and punishment:

> Since promiscuity of the types which lead to V.D. is seldom the result of positive mature interest but mainly the result of attempts to relieve acute psychological stress, neither punishment on the one hand nor evil counsel on the other is likely to affect to any marked degree the incidence of such promiscuity.

Indeed, a program of fear may place the medical officer in the awkward position of providing reassurance to the patient he is treating, when he has previously terrified the soldier with the potential consequences of venereal infection. This fear is not only useless in preventing exposure to infection, but it magnifies the problems of hypochondriasis and neurosis following exposure.

It is well documented that the venereal disease rate reflects leadership and consequent morale within a military unit.[13-17] The responsibility for unit morale rests with the leader, depending upon his ability to gain rapport with his troops and to understand human behavior. These qualities are often deficient in the army officer. His authority is usually guaranteed by his rank rather than by his personality or qualities of understanding and leadership. Nevertheless, the personal example of the officers themselves is of great importance. Dunham,[18] a former general of the U.S. Army Medical Corps, considered that the company commander was of key importance because his attitudes will be reflected in the actions of his men. Sensational or illogical statements by him do vastly more harm than good. Rather than alleviate the problems by setting a good example, officers frequently aggravate low morale by lack of consideration for their men. Stouffer[19] has expressed the view, in general terms, that men will accept hardship with complacency if they realize that nothing can be done about it, but they become angry and disgruntled when some personnel, especially officers, get more than their share of scarce goods and privileges. This facet of poor management was utilized as propaganda to reduce the morale of Communist terrorists in Malaya,

> Too never lost an opportunity of telling the truth about women in the jungle, who inevitably became mistresses of the higher-ranking officers—an aspect of jungle life that infuriated thousands of C.T.s, who had to watch their officers taking mistresses while the rank and file could not.[20]

Moralistic counsel of abstinence for the troops, while officers continue to frequent brothels or openly take mistresses, is likely to have an adverse impact on unit morale and increase the incidence of venereal infection.

As part of a restrictive policy in coping with venereal disease, the military usually attempts to restrict access of soldiers to the prostitutes who are inevitably attracted by aggregations of troops. Declaring certain areas out-of-bounds or off limits is one component of this policy. The task of implementing this policy, however, is doomed to failure. As one American medical officer wrote:

> As a preventive-medical officer in Vietnam, I watched the V.D. rate stay at a high level despite efforts to control the sources. Even nightly Military Police patrols have failed to keep "off-limit" areas GI free. If such efforts have worked in previous military conflicts, be advised that this one is thus different in still another way.[21]

No matter how closely soldiers are supervised or restricted, it is not practically possible to separate them from sexual partners. One soldier acquired VD within days of his arrival in Vietnam when he alighted from a leading vehicle in a slow-moving convoy, had intercourse on the roadside, and rejoined the convoy on a vehicle further to the rear. Others would stop on the roadside or at roadside cafes and engage in hurried intercourse or fellatio before continuing their journey. Faced with this outlook and behavior, the task of denying opportunity for sex to such soldiers is a formidable, if not impossible, one. On their part, the prostitutes gained entry to camps disguised as "sandbaggers," patients in ambulances, or domestic staff. Others moved into the countryside to seduce the troops at work, and intercourse occurred on the roadside. The off-limits policy fails, as do many other control policies, because it is no match for the combined ingenuity of the prostitutes and their prospective clients that always triumphs over any barrier to their union.

Control policies which recur in wartime include mass prostitute examination and testing and the organized brothel. The shortcomings of both these policies have been fully discussed in Chapter 5. The natural difficulties inherent in enforced examination of prostitutes are compounded in wartime when untrained or partially-trained staff are used for collecting and interpreting laboratory samples, and the overall screening program is conducted by nonmedical personnel. The concept of the organized brothel ignores two key features of wartime sexual behavior. First, the task of providing for the sexual outlet of even 100,000 troops in wartime is a formidable one clearly beyond the capability of any one organization. Secondly, the greater part of sexual activity in wartime is of an impromptu nature, occurring spontaneously in response to prostitute seduction or sudden impulse, in some cases influenced by alcohol or peer encouragement. These participants would not contemplate visiting a brothel that was explicitly allocated for sexual indulgence. Many other soldiers would be discouraged by the formality and regimentation involved in an organized military brothel.

The inadequacies of military control policies are aggravated by the involvement of combat officers and the military police. These officers often devise and maintain control programs with only superficial involvement of medical personnel. Consequently, such programs usually involve systems which have repeatedly proven to be failures or which are medically unsound. Furthermore, personal involvement and corruption are inevitably associated with these schemes. Even when they are initiated with the purest motives, they soon degenerate into convenient social and sexual outlets for the officers and their friends. This situation, even when carefully disguised, is easily recognized by the troop population and only serves to lower morale.

The outlook for venereal disease control is not always so pessimistic. In certain circumstances remarkable results may be achieved, particularly where both the troop and prostitute populations are static and are isolated from outside influence. Greenberg[11] has described the success of unauthorized regulation of prostitutes in Korea:

> In one small isolated detachment in Korea the venereal disease rate was maintained at a genuine zero for a long period of time because the girls in the neighboring village were examined and treated regularly by the detachment surgeon. As there was no transient population there was almost no opportunity for the introduction of venereal disease.

The environments where intervention is appropriate and the best control methods to be used, however, can only be assessed by a venereologist with experience of military conditions.

The impact of venereal disease on military populations can be greatly reduced, but this will never be achieved unless there is a radical change in military policy. Venereal disease is a complex medicosocial problem. Its control should be under the direction of a competent venereologist.

Obsessive preoccupation with venereal disease incidence serves no useful purpose. The interpretation of venereal disease statistics is difficult for a venereologist and is clearly beyond the comprehension of a military officer. In many situations, a high incidence of venereal infection must be accepted. Even when reduction is possible, the manpower and resources required to achieve this result may outweigh the benefits obtained. It is more appropriate to view venereal infection as merely a manifestation of maladjustment in a stressful situation. The rational approach to this problem requires action that will assist the individual in coping with stress. The combat officer can assist by developing close rapport with his troops so that he is aware of their grievances and can take appropriate remedial action. Stress is very much a subjective phenomenon. It can only be alleviated by consideration of the attitudes and feelings of the individuals experiencing it. Often the knowledge that someone genuinely cares and is attempting to improve their conditions improves troop morale even if no material benefits eventuate.

Seamen

"The traveller par excellence is the merchant seaman and, by reason of his calling, he is more exposed to temptation than those of other occupations."[22]

Among seamen, the sociological background responsible for venereal infection has much in common with that of the military. The seaman is confronted with harsh living conditions, loneliness, and enforced absence from family and homeland. He lives exclusively among men, often has a monotonous daily routine, and has little opportunity for a normal sex life. This life inevitably takes its toll on the individual.

Poor living quarters in ship or ashore, boredom through lack of interesting recreation, or a lack of group morale owing to unjust discipline or conditions of work, may induce a rebellious spirit which results in a deterioration of individual character.[22]

By comparison with these conditions, arrival in a port and access to its women, no matter how squalid, provides welcome relief. Realizing this demand for their services, prostitutes and casually promiscuous females congregate around the wharves and adjacent hotels of most seaports. Consequently these ports tend to have a high venereal disease incidence, a high proportion of which can be traced to sailors. Of 400 consecutive cases of infection seen in Liverpool, 94 were local men, 58 from elsewhere in the British Isles, and 248 from overseas. Over 75 percent of the overseas men compared to only 13 percent of the Liverpool men, were infected by a prostitute.[22]

The problem is aggravated by the mobility of sailors and the anonymous nature of many of their contacts. Contact tracing is virtually impossible in many cases. In a 1948 study, 80 unselected seafarers admitted intercourse with 615 persons in 112 ports in 45 different countries.[23]

Additional distress was caused at a personal level by the difficulties in obtaining adequate treatment in foreign lands. This was alleviated by the Brussels agreement, which was signed in 1924. Briefly, the signatories to this agreement undertook to establish and maintain in principal ports services for the free treatment of venereal disease in seamen of all nationalities. Each patient received a personal card, designated by a number only, enabling some continuity of management.

A much greater impact has been made by a change in the social conditions of seamen. Due to containerization and other modern techniques, there are relatively fewer seamen. These mostly enjoy reasonable living conditions. Due to the increased speed of modern ships and other communications, seamen are away from home for shorter periods, receive more regular mail from their families, and generally feel less isolated from normal social relationships. Consequently, the relative contribution of seamen to the overall problem of venereal disease control is declining, and this trend is likely to continue. This decline offers an example showing that greater gains in venereal disease control are made by solving the fundamental social problems responsible for infection than by attacking the isolated manifestations of these problems.

Individuals Who Do Not Contract Venereal Disease

By comparison with VD patients, we know very little of the psychological and behavioral characteristics of individuals who do not contract venereal disease. In a way, focus on VD patients represents a negative approach. These patients represent the failure rather than the success of preventive measures. Closer study of the non-VD group may reveal unknown prophylactic features and may provide a more accurate assessment of those measures which have been investigated among VD patients. As venereal infection is so strongly dependent on promiscuity, it follows that the non-VD group consists of a) those who are not promiscuous and b) those who are promiscuous but who manage to escape the sequelae attendant on others who behave in similar manner. It is this latter group, in particular, that warrants closer study. Obviously, if VD patients utilized the same prophylatic measures (in the most general sense) of their uninfected counterparts, the incidence of venereal disease would be greatly reduced. This is of real practical significance. Behavior specifically involved in preventing infection is more amenable to modification than the underlying forces resulting in promiscuity.

Some VD patients who are reluctant to alter their sexual behavior are eager to avoid infection or other unpleasant results from this behavior. We need to know in precise detail why some individuals who indulge in the same sexual behavior as others contract venereal disease while the others apparently do not.

Chapter Eleven

Failure to Control
Venereal Disease

Although statistics suggest that the incidence of venereal infection is increasing, the extent of this increase is uncertain. Due to administrative difficulties, limited reporting by physicians, and clandestine treatment or nontreatment, official statistics represent only a small proportion of the true incidence. While this proportion may be 10 percent or less in developed countries it is even lower in more primitive communities where statistics may reveal only 1 percent of infections. With improved venereology services and increased patient and physician cooperation, a marked improvement in reporting may be expected. Screening programs may also disclose many cases of infection that otherwise would remain undetected.

Certain demographic features may also give a false impression of control over venereal disease. Even if the rate of infection remains the same, more cases can be expected from an increasing population. Particularly in developing countries, urban growth rates may increase 50 percent–100 percent in a decade. It has already been suggested that urban populations create greater VD problems than rural ones (see Chapter 10). In 1971, Oslo had 13 percent of the population but had 36.3 percent of the new cases of gonorrhea and syphilis in Norway. In 1970, Paris, with 5.7 percent of the population, contributed 50 percent of gonorrhea and 43 percent of early syphilis to French statistics.

In 1969–1970, Colombo, with only 4.8 percent of the population, produced more than 60 percent of the early syphilis and gonorrhea in Ceylon.[1] These figures may, of course, merely represent better communications and reporting in the urban centers from which epidemiologic control is directed.

Regardless of the real trend in VD incidence, however, the actual incidence is obviously so great and present methods so limited in impact, there can be little doubt that venereal disease is uncontrolled. Many factors contributing to this failure have been suggested, but a critical analysis of these factors is important in order to establish some measure of the relative importance of each factor to the overall problem. Some of these play a dominant role in the shortcomings of control policies, others are less important, and some are trivial or of theoretical interest only. Some of these dubious influences, such as the introduction of the pill and venereal disease education, have already been discussed.

Complacency

The interest in venereal disease during recent years was preceded by a long period of complacency among administrators, physicians, and the general public. The advent of penicillin and other antibiotics removed the fear of venereal infection. Many considered control was a foregone conclusion. Against this background, concealment and gross underreporting of venereal disease allowed the surreptitious dissemination of the infection to produce the enormous present-day incidence. This phenomenon might be termed primary complacency, *i.e.*, failure to appreciate the existence of the problem.

In some communities, mobilization of the available sources controlled and reduced venereal infection to a point where at least temporary eradication was in sight. This situation was achieved in syphilis control in the United States in the 1950s. At this point, there was excessive reduction of funds for venereal disease services, clinics were closed, and medical attention was diverted elsewhere. The inevitable resurgence of syphilis followed. This might be termed secondary complacency, *i.e.*, a delusion that the problem has been solved.

At the present time some impact is being made on primary complacency. Administrators and physicians in many countries are acknowledging the problem and are offering at least verbal support for its solution. If venereal disease is again controlled in the future, there will be a tendency for withdrawal of this hard-earned support and the problem will resume. There can be little doubt that complete control of venereal disease requires persistent vigilance with a constant outlay of personnel and resources.

Treatment Facilities

Complacency and consequent lack of finance has precluded the provision of sufficient VD clinics; however, the nature of existing clinics has had more far-reaching consequences. As most public clinics are often squalid, ill-equipped, and poorly staffed, it is not surprising that many patients are treated privately. In practice, this excludes epidemiologic investigation of a high proportion of cases.

These clinics have set the whole tone of venereology and have created a uniformly poor image among the public and the medical profession. Not only have they discouraged the attendance of many patients and restricted the cooperation of others but they have also prevented the recruitment of high-quality medical graduates and paramedical staff to the field of venereology. The indirect impact resulting from this image of venereology is as important as that resulting from the poor therapeutic facilities provided.

Influence of the Medical Profession

Venereal disease has been virtually ignored by medical schools throughout the world. This explains the apparent paradox that contagious urethritis, the most common disease seen by physicians and one of the easiest to diagnose and treat effectively is, in fact, managed less adequately than most other conditions. Space does not permit a catalog of even the more gross blunders perpetrated by practicing physicians, nor would this serve any useful purpose. In general terms, it may be said that the average physician has difficulty in distinguishing among contagious nongonococcal urethritis, gonorrhea, and noncontagious urethritis. He fails to appreciate the need for highly specific antibiotic treatment of gonorrhea. He is unaware that only a few antibiotics are effective for treating nongonococcal urethritis and that even these have only a limited role in the management of this condition.

Inadequacies in the psychosocial and epidemiologic management of patients are the most disturbing features, however. The hesitancy and uncertainty of the doctor are readily transmitted to the patient, and inadequate treatment soon declares itself. These shortcomings aggravate, rather than alleviate the anxieties and neuroses that are so intimately involved with venereal infection. The physician usually complicates instead of simplifying the social sequelae of infection. An incorrect diagnosis of venereal infection, in particular, with its social implications, exposes the doctor to legal prosecution as well as reflecting technical incompetence.

It is essential that physicians should not be unduly criticized at a personal level for their management of venereal disease. This is unlikely to remedy the situation or to enlist their future cooperation. Venereologists should adopt a sympathetic approach, provide essential information whenever possible, and assure the general practitioner that advice and support are available on request at any time. The primary solution to inadequate medical information resides with the medical schools, which are directly responsible for providing at least a rudimentary knowledge of the more important diseases occurring in the community. This cannot be achieved without providing venereology posts in residency and intern training as well as offering instruction in the undergraduate program.

Public Attitudes

The restraining influences of religion, family, and public opinion have diminished; promiscuity is viewed less unfavorably than in the past. Shame and guilt and consequent reluctance to acknowledge infection are nevertheless still major features of the venereal diseases. This reticence hinders epidemiologic investigation, particularly where nonvaginal coitus is involved.

Specific attitudes to venereal disease, however, are greatly influenced by the attitudes of the medical profession and the nature and conduct of treatment clinics. Certainly young people have a healthier attitude toward sexuality and its sequelae than preceding generations. If the medical profession places its own house in order, future public attitudes should provide little hindrance to venereal disease control.

Female Reservoir of Infection

"The primary reason for the high incidence of venereal disease in U.S. troops is, as it has been in Korea and elsewhere, the large uncontrolled, infected prostitute population."[2]

This is undoubtedly so in Asia where 80 percent–90 percent of VD is acquired from prostitutes. This proportion is much less in most Western countries and, with the increase in promiscuity for pleasure, is likely to decline even further. As Willcox[3] states, "The key is not prostitution, but promiscuity in both sexes." It is the promiscuous pool of infection which renders control so difficult. Gonococcal infection in females is usually asymptomatic, difficult to diagnose, and is usually disclosed by contact tracing.

The concept of the asymptomatic female pool as representing the total problem is a gross oversimplification. Present evidence suggests that asymptomatic infection in the male may be almost as significant. Although only a small proportion (probably less than 3 percent) of infected men remain asymptomatic, these accumulate in the community as the symptomatic men are treated and removed from the infected pool. Consequently, the prevalence of asymptomatic infection in infected men at any one time may reach 50 percent. A further problem is that many symptomatic individuals do not readily seek treatment. They may not be aware of the significance of their symptoms, or they may be reluctant to seek treatment because of the location of the health provider, financial considerations, the attitude and behavior of health providers, delays in being treated, the interviewing process, the type of care they receive, or ill-defined attitudes of their own. The infected pool, therefore, consists of a diverse group of individuals, both men and women, both symptomatic and asymptomatic.

The problem is to identify and treat these individuals soon after they have become infected. At present this cannot be achieved in many communities. Contact tracing is expensive, time consuming, and at best locates only a limited portion of the pool. A suitable serologic test for gonorrhea would provide a more acceptable alternative to vaginal examination for screening large populations, but it would have a limited role in control, as evidenced by syphilis dissemination. An increasing awareness of asymptomatic infection, particularly in men, and an appreciation of the personal value of treatment are encouraging many promiscuous individuals to seek routine testing. This is clearly a desirable trend.

Lomholt and Berg[4] suggested treating, on the same day, all patients acquiring gonorrhea within the past 6 months and all single persons between 16 and 29. This may be practicable in small, isolated, cooperative communities but is unlikely to have widespread application.

Population Mobility

The increasing mobility of the world population poses one of the major challenges to venereal disease control. The *Wall Street Journal* account of a California prostitute with syphilis illustrates the problem created by this mobility. Among her contacts, 168 long-distance truck drivers were traced. Subsequent to contact, these men had traveled over

34 American states, Canada, and Mexico.[5] With modern travel, the problems once confined to the armed forces, seamen, and commercial travelers now involve a large proportion of the total population.

The likelihood of locating sexual contacts is directly related to the distance they have traveled after contact. In one study[6] the proportions of contacts located in the same city, 500–1000 miles away, 1000–2000 miles away, and more than 2000 miles away from the patient were 81 percent, 63 percent, 57 percent, and 44 percent respectively. The syphilis yield from those examined was approximately 15/100 in all groups. Not only is the total yield reduced by present-day mobility, but the cost of locating each contact is greatly increased.

High-Risk Groups

Certain high-risk groups have been discussed. Clearly the best returns might be expected from those groups which contribute disproportionately to the venereal disease incidence. The identification of these groups is an important part of control in any community. Conversely, failure to identify these groups or to demonstrate their absence will decrease the efficiency of any program. While these groups are often defined in terms of sociological parameters, locality may be the most important feature. Certain hotels or residential areas may constitute important foci of infection. It is essential to realize that control will be facilitated by eradicating the infection from these foci but without disrupting the underlying social structure within the foci. Oppressive measures against the participants in these areas, with involvement of the police and other institutions, will only scatter the infected participants who will take up a variety of clandestine activities. This will make control much more difficult, if not impossible.

Immunization

Immunization has transformed the control of many infections. Despite an initial burst of enthusiasm in which some individuals saw immunization as the conqueror of all infectious disease, subsequent experience has demonstrated that this epidemiologic tool has a highly variable contribution to make to the control of different diseases. Reluctantly the limitations of even some vaccines with international use, such as cholera, are being recognized. The more important factors influencing the value of a particular vaccine include its effectiveness, the risk and severity of side-effects, the risk and severity of the disease, and patient acceptance or administrative enforcement.

The likely role of vaccination for venereal disease must be assessed against this background. The most effective vaccines have been developed for disease conditions that of themselves confer lifetime or long-standing immunity—a property of neither syphilis nor gonorrhea. The epidemiologic role of vaccination is greatest for diseases for which other prophylactic procedures are limited, adequate definitive treatment is not available, or severe sequelae occur despite treatment. For gonorrhea and syphilis adequate prophylaxis and simple highly effective treatment are available. One of the most severe limitations of vaccination programs is shared with venereal disease control—both depend greatly on attitudes and prejudices. The general population is not particularly receptive to epidemiologic control as evidenced by the low acceptance rate of many voluntary vaccination programs (polio being a notable exception). It is only due to enforcement that high rates are obtained in such groups as overseas travelers, school children, and the armed forces. With the added stigma attached to venereal infection, it is difficult to imagine the population flocking to vaccination centers for venereal disease.

If an effective vaccine were developed, it would have a definite role among those few individuals who are repeated attenders at VD clinics, but otherwise it would have limited impact. The failure to control venereal disease is not due to a lack of scientific aids in prevention and treatment but to our lack of understanding and influence over human behavior. For this reason, it is unlikely that vaccination will play a significant role in controlling venereal infection in the near future.

Chapter Twelve

Controlling Venereal Infection

Few areas of medical practice have suffered from bureaucratic obstruction to a greater extent than venereal disease control. In both military and civilian environments, high-quality physicians have been reluctant to take an interest in this field. Programs have often been designed and implemented by an array of unqualified personnel, often with no medical training and only minimal knowledge of infectious diseases. Such programs have developed in diverse directions, but they all share a common feature—failure to control venereal disease.

In some areas, authorities have practiced intellectual escapism by putting emphasis on meetings or committees that frequently make theoretical or philosophic recommendations without regard to practicability or likelihood of eventual implementation. The Federal Coordinating Committee in Australia that was formed in 1965[1] to investigate the problem of venereal disease illustrates such an approach. Included in the fifteen members of this committee were representatives of the Catholic Welfare Bureau, the Salvation Army, the Australian Council of Churches, police departments, the armed forces, the Commonwealth Office of Education, the Australian Council of Social Service, and one venereologist. The report of this committee, though technically of little relevance, did contain fifteen recommendations. These recommendations have made little, if any, impact on venereology in Australia in the past 10 years. Most of them have been partially or totally ignored. At a time when many countries are considering international cooperative measures, there is still no national coordinating body in Australia.

Other programs have developed large complex organizations making considerable expenditures to implement practical policies. The control techniques employed have never been adequately evaluated, however, and thus the reason for their evident failure is unknown. In these organizations, the bureaucratic machine which has evolved may be resistant to innovation and may act as a barrier to the introduction of different epidemiologic techniques that have potential for success.

In any area, control is unlikely unless the medical profession, the public, and the government agree on the priority of the problem, and are prepared to cooperate in providing the funds, facilities, staff, and research necessary for its solution. Available resources must be utilized with maximum efficiency. Priorities must be established for control procedures, and these must be subjected to cost–benefit analysis.

This chapter outlines a sequential program for venereal disease control. Each component should be developed to reasonable sophistication before introducing the next, rather than spreading available resources over a number of poorly developed components.

Plan or Control Program

Specialized Coordinating Staff

Venereal disease control is difficult and requires a highly specialized knowledge of clinical medicine, epidemiology, and sociology. It is unlikely that the average medical practitioner has greater expertise in this field than in any other medical specialty in which he has not had specific training; in practice, because of the long-standing neglect of venereology in medical teaching, the medical profession tends to have a specific ignorance in this field. It is quite inappropriate for venereal disease control policy to be decided by representatives from sundry medical fields. It is therefore essential that those who direct or coordinate any program have a sound training and background in the epidemiology of infectious diseases, with particular emphasis on the venereal diseases.

Clinical Services

Without effective diagnosis and treatment, other aids to control, no matter how sophisticated, are largely wasted. The establishment of specialized clinics with an attached laboratory for the management of patients and for the provision of support to other physicians and facilities in the region has top priority.

Figure 12-1 shows the design and staffing of a clinic capable of acting as a control center for venereal disease in a particular area. The laboratory of this center should be able to perform all the routine tests for venereal disease. This service should be available for all clinicians in the area of control. Figure 12-2 shows one method of expanding this basic design to enable the clinic to fulfill a teaching role. For large clinics a simple operating suite to cope with simple surgical procedures may be warranted. Availability of either staff or personnel may necessitate appropriate modification of either clinic design.

Documentation should be tailored to meet the needs of an individual clinic, but there are three essential components for effective individual management. The first of these is the individual case record. Figure 12-3 shows one example of an individual case record. This has a simple format and allows a ready check on the treatment or surveillance status of the patient. A section of the record to summarize attendances is useful, particularly for recidivists whose records often become lengthy and complex. Male and female case records are best differentiated by the use of different colored paper. Secondly, there should be a register of daily attendance, which is useful for statistical compilations. It may also be used as an appointment book. Also, an alphabetical register of patients is particularly helpful for locating case records if these are stored in different locations (depending on the treatment status of the patient), or if they are not stored alphabetically. A simple procedure for a check on defaulting can be incorporated into any one of these components. Data for research purposes should be collected and collated independently from the documents used for individual management.

Apart from the therapeutic treatment of established, bacteriologically proven infection, three other types of treatment are often employed in venereology—prophylactic, abortive, and epidemiologic. As these terms are frequently misused and their application even more frequently abused, a brief consideration of their roles is warranted.

Prophylactic treatment refers to an antibiotic administered prior to exposure for the express purpose of preventing infection.

Abortive treatment refers to an antibiotic administered after exposure for the express purpose of aborting the clinical manifestations of any infection that may have been acquired. Although a smaller quantity of antibiotic is required to eradicate preclinical infection, there is

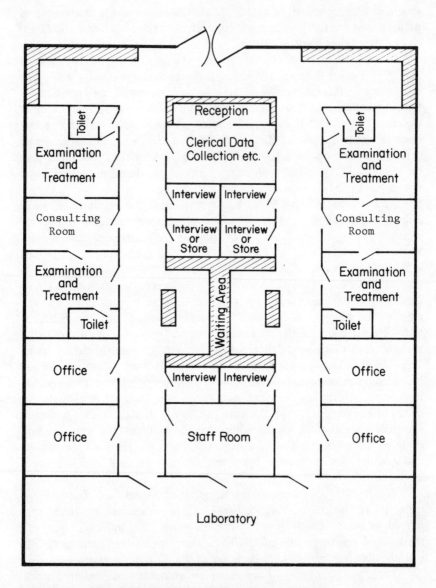

FIGURE 12–1 VENEREAL DISEASE CLINIC (control center)
Design and Staffing

Capability: 20 patients/hour (Including surveillance patients)
Staff: Medical Director, 2 Medical Officers, 4 Clinical Assistants, 4 Case Find-
ers, Receptionist/Clerk, Secretary, and 5 Laboratory Assistants

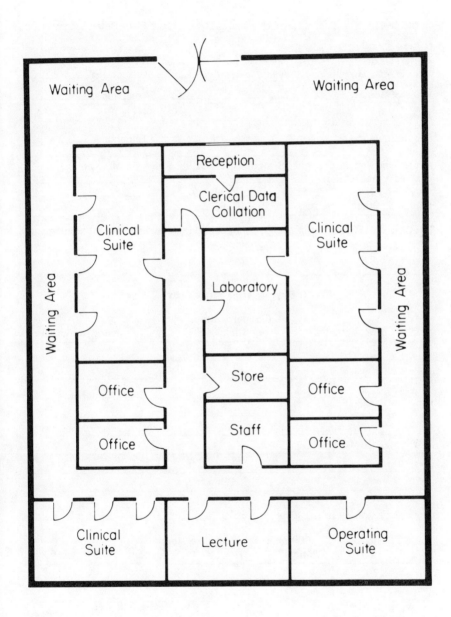

FIGURE 12–2 VENEREAL DISEASE CLINIC AND TEACHING UNIT

FIGURE 12-3 PERSONAL CASE RECORD
Clinic Number

Surname _____ Given name _____ Birth Date _____
                          (inc. nickname) _____

Marital status   Country of origin _____
   S   M   W   D   Sep.   (years in country) _____ Occupation _____

Place of work _____ Telephone _____

Address _____ Telephone _____

Contacting address _____ Telephone _____

Reason for first attendance: Symptoms; Exposure; Referral—MO, Clinic,
contact, other; Other: _____
Previous VD: _____
Allergies, Other illnesses: _____

SPECIAL NOTES: e.g., prophylaxis, contraception, problems of sexual adjustment

----

ATTENDANCE SUMMARY

		Clinical features		
Date	Investigations	or Diagnosis	Treatment	Other

Clinical Notes (reverse side)

Date	Clinical	Investigations	Sig/next visit

always a risk that small doses will merely mask clinical manifestations without eradicating the organism. For this reason, full therapeutic dosage must be used for any form of treatment (including the prophylactic and abortive). No single drug protects against all sexually transmitted disease, and any proponent of these treatments must choose between multidrug admininstration with consequent increased risk of side-effects or providing only partial protection at best.

Epidemiologic treatment refers to an antibiotic administered when a diagnosis of an established infection is accepted on epidemiologic grounds before the results of confirmatory diagnostic tests are known. This is discussed more fully in the next section.

Epidemiology of Control

Although some health workers use the term venereal disease epidemiology as synonymous with contact tracing, this usage is confusing and should be discontinued. Epidemiology has been defined in many ways, but certainly it refers to the distribution and determinants of disease in a community. The epidemiology of venereal disease consists of all those factors—clinical, bacteriologic, and sociological—that produce the spectrum of and influence the control of the diseases in the community.

The epidemiologist must develop an intimate knowledge of the dynamics of disease dissemination. From this knowledge he must implement the intervention program to which the transmission is most susceptible. The epidemiology of venereal disease involves the disease, the environment, and the host (Figure 12-4).

Disease. The personal and community impact of each disease differs, and its individual management and epidemic control must be considered separately. In Figure 12-4, the venereal diseases have been arranged, somewhat arbitrarily, according to the relative role of sexual transmission in their dissemination. Although many cases of scabies and pediculosis are transmitted sexually, the majority of cases result from close nonsexual contact. At the other extreme, sexual intimacy is the dominant factor in the transmission of gonorrhea. For comparison, candidiasis and hepatitis B have been included.

The contribution of sexual transmission to the total morbidity of hepatitis B is still uncertain. Similar uncertainty exists for group B streptococcal infection. Whereas *Candida* may be transmitted sexually, this transmission makes only slight contribution to the total disease morbidity. *Candida* is a commensal organism, and its pathogenic impact is largely determined by concurrent systemic illness, hormonal balance, bacterial imbalance (often affected by broad spectrum anti-

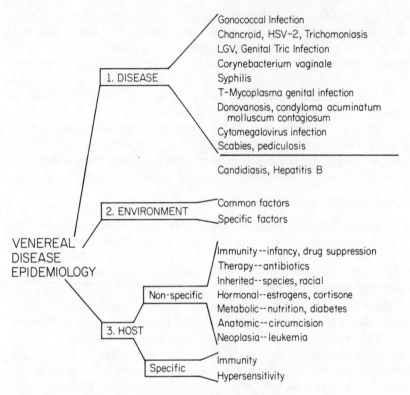

FIGURE 12–4 EPIDEMIOLOGY OF VENEREAL DISEASE

biotics), and local factors influencing surface moisture and integrity. Classification as a venereal disease is consequently inappropriate.

Environment. There may be little similarity between the epidemiology of a disease in one environment and that of the same disease in another environment. Although findings from other areas offer general guidelines to the relevant factors involved, the epidemiology of each condition must be investigated independently in each environment. This is best illustrated by the transmission of gonorrhea.

Common features of gonorrhea epidemiology include transmission in an erratic fashion by coitus. The chance of transmission from an infected female is less than 50 percent. From an infected male it is more than 50 percent. In most men there is a short incubation period before the disease becomes established. The disease is usually symptomatic in males and asymptomatic in females. Gonococcal infection of pharynx or rectum may occur from homosexual or heterosexual contact, and these infections are usually asymptomatic.

Gonorrhea is not randomly distributed in the population, however. Control depends on determination of the high-risk groups, discovering the mechanism underlying their increased risk, and assessing the available methods of eliminating the disease from these groups. It should be kept in mind that this distribution and its underlying mechanism as well as the feasibility of control may differ markedly from one environment to another. The quantitation of these factors provides the specific features of gonorrhea epidemiology.

Figure 12-5 shows a simplified cycle of gonorrhea transmission, indicating some of the contributions to the infected pool. There are many steps in the management process. At each step, some infected individuals are lost from the curative process and accumulate in the infected pool. Clearly for effective control this fallout must be minimized, and it may be helpful for controllers to monitor each component of the process individually.

Figure 12-6 outlines common types of exposure producing gonococcal infections. While there is a general tendency for symptomatic individuals to receive treatment and for asymptomatic individuals to escape it, some symptomatic patients do not seek treatment, whereas screening and contact tracing do locate significant numbers of asymptomatic but infected individuals. The net effect of this process produces a high proportion of asymptomatic infection in the residual pool. This pool also contains many symptomatic individuals of both sexes, including those with infections of the pharynx and rectum as well as those with urethral or endocervical infection. The relative contribution of each component to the total pool will vary with many factors. The balance of homosexual and heterosexual outlets and the type of sexual practices indulged in in a particular community should particularly be noted.

Figure 12-7 outlines some of the more important parameters influencing disease control. For a rational approach to disease control, the parameters listed in these figures must be quantitated and the reason for their contribution understood.

Host factors. Host factors may be specific (influencing only one infection) or nonspecific (influencing most infections).

Sensitivity and Specificity

Sensitivity is the percentage of positive results in a series of specimens taken from patients who actually have the disease. Specificity is

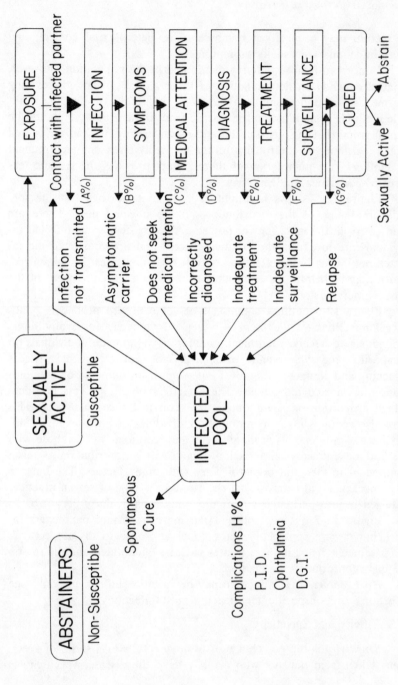

FIGURE 12-5 SIMPLIFIED CYCLE OF GONORRHEA TRANSMISSION

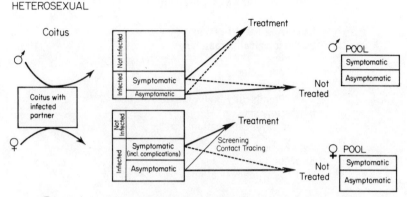

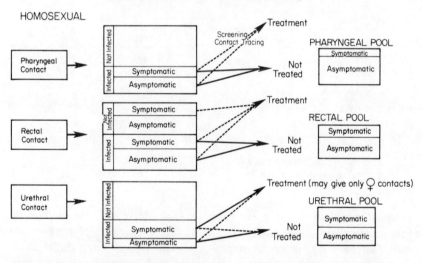

FIGURE 12–6 COMMON TYPES OF SEXUAL EXPOSURE (Exposure and symptoms for gonorrhea)

the percentage of negative results in a series of specimens taken from normal subjects who do not have the disease considered. These concepts may be clarified by considering the results of a screening study put in the form depicted in Figure 12-8.

It is important that screening tests for venereal disease be highly sensitive; confirmatory diagnostic tests must be highly specific. The utility of a test is also dependent on the prevalence of disease in the

FIGURE 12-7   IMPORTANT PARAMETERS INFLUENCING INFECTIOUS DISEASE CONTROL

1. Localizing Identification
   2. Sociological parameters
      Age
      Education
      Race
      Promiscuity including Prostitution
   b. Recidivism
   c. Geographical location

2. Ease of Detection
   a. Mobility
   b. Ease of identification

FIGURE 12-8   CLASSIFICATION OF SCREENING RESULTS

Test Results	Diagnosis		Total
	Diseased	Not Diseased	
Positive	a	b	a + b
Negative	c	d	c + d
Total	a + c	b + d	a + b + c + d

From this data $\text{Sensitivity} = \dfrac{a}{a + c} \times 100$

$\text{Specificity} = \dfrac{d}{b + d} \times 100$

b = false positives to the test
c = false negative to the test

sampled population. As prevalence (a + c) decreases, the impact of false-positive results increases, *i.e.*, a smaller proportion of positive results [a / (a + b)] come from patients who actually have the disease. Treponemal tests often perform very well because they are used on sera that have already proven positive with reagin tests, *i.e.*, populations of very high disease prevalence. They may perform poorly, however, when used for screening of populations whose disease prevalence is low.

These principles can be illustrated by comparing a reagin test (R) of 95 percent sensitivity and 90 percent specificity with a treponemal test (S) of 99 percent sensitivity and 99 percent specificity. In a population with a syphilis prevalence of 10 percent, each 1000 individuals will contain 100 with syphilis and 900 without. The use of R for screening and S for confirmation (on positives from R) yields the following results:

	Positive R	Positive S
100 with syphilis	95	94
900 without syphilis	90	1

There will be positive R tests in 48.6 percent [90 / (90 + 95)] of the patients without syphilis. Only 1 percent [1 / (95 + 1)] of positive S patients are without disease. If S is used for screening, however, it will be positive for 99 patients with disease and 9 without disease; 8.3 percent [9 / (99 + 9)] of positive tests occur in patients without disease.

Incidence and Prevalence

The epidemiology of venereal disease cannot be assessed adequately without a clear understanding of the concepts of prevalence and incidence and the relationship between these two parameters. *Incidence* is defined as the number of new cases of infection occurring in a given time interval. *Prevalence* is the number of cases of infection in a community at any moment in time or during a particular specified time period. Clearly the relationship between incidence and prevalence is directly related to the duration of illness. Under stable disease conditions,

$$\text{Prevalence} = \text{Incidence} \times \text{Duration.}$$

Chronic conditions with low incidence will have a relatively high prevalence. This difference contributes to the disagreement over the relative contribution of asymptomatic gonorrhea in the male. Asymptomatic gonorrhea probably accounts for 1–3 percent of all male gonococcal infections. However, the symptomatic cases are treated early and have a short duration, whereas asymptomatic cases remain undetected and accumulate in the population. Screening of males, particularly if selected groups are chosen, may reveal that 20–50 percent of those with gonococcal infection are asymptomatic. These divergent proportions do not provide conflicting evidence of the frequency of asymptomatic infection but merely demonstrate that it has a low incidence (1–3 percent) but a high prevalence (20–50 percent) among infected males.

Prevalence of a disease has important implications for serological screening. With low prevalence, the small return of cases does not justify the expense involved. Furthermore, the impact of false positives increases (as discussed above).

Disease Control

"The answer is that it is easier to modify a health program than it is to change the population."[2]

The control of animal disease has been facilitated by the thoroughness with which sanctions can be employed. Bovine contagious pleuropneumonia, glanders, foot-and-mouth disease, and dourine (a venereal disease of horses) were all controlled by slaughter of infected animals. Rabies was eradicated from England in 1896 by the enforced muzzling of all dogs for a one-year period.

Such aggressive measures cannot be used in human disease. Figure 12-9 outlines, in general terms, alternate pathways to disease control. Clinicobacterial expertise alone is never adequate for control, for the fullest potential of these techniques cannot be attained without the cooperation of the community at risk. Individuals are usually reluctant to restrict their personal behavior or cooperate uniformly, and success in controlling human disease has usually resulted from epidemiologic expertise, frequently with the imposition of control sanctions.

Manipulation of disease environment. This is among the major approaches to disease control. A reticulated water supply and a unified sewerage system provide the definitive counter to cholera and most other enteric diseases. Diseases mediated by vectors are often most efficiently controlled by a concerted effort directed against one component of the transmission chain. Rat control is an important element of antiplague campaigns. Anti-mite measures provide significant benefit against typhus. The mosquito is probably the most significant vector of infectious disease. Despite enormous expenditure on personnel and resources, success in disrupting transmission through this medium has been variable.

Although this type of control is often the most effective, in most situations it is inapplicable to any of the venereal diseases. In some environments, a segregated prostitute population may provide the sole sexual outlet for a male community. If infection is eliminated from this prostitute group, which is only possible when the women are segregated from other contact, modification of male behavior patterns (a more difficult task requiring constant monitoring) is not required. This technique was used to eradicate venereal disease from one group of American troops during the Korean war.[3]

Quarantine. Quarantine has been widely and effectively used, particularly for diseases for which no adequate therapy exists. Placing areas off-limits to soldiers has been used by the military for centuries, but it has never been any match for the combined ingenuity of prosti-

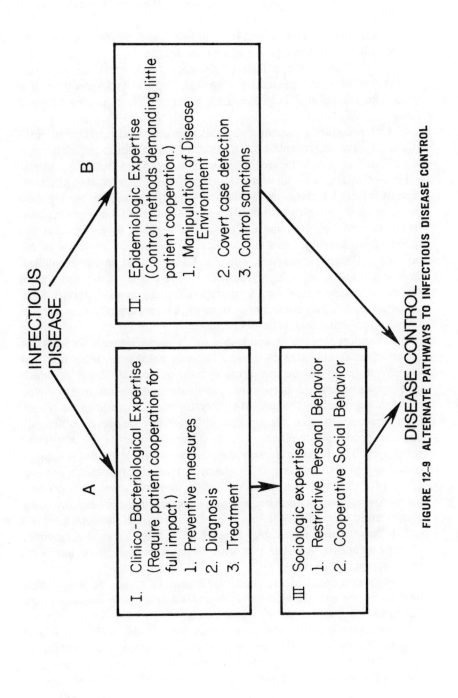

INFECTIOUS DISEASE

A

B

I. Clinico-Bacteriological Expertise
(Require patient cooperation for full impact.)
1. Preventive measures
2. Diagnosis
3. Treatment

II. Epidemiologic Expertise
(Control methods demanding little patient cooperation.)
1. Manipulation of Disease Environment
2. Covert case detection
3. Control sanctions

III Sociologic expertise
1. Restrictive Personal Behavior
2. Cooperative Social Behavior

DISEASE CONTROL

FIGURE 12-9 ALTERNATE PATHWAYS TO INFECTIOUS DISEASE CONTROL

tutes and soldiers. This principle is unlikely to have any applicability in controlling venereal disease in civilian society.

Prophylaxis. The principle of prophylaxis refers to voluntary acceptance of some preventive technique before exposure to a disease. The two most widely used techniques are chemoprophylaxis and immunoprophylaxis.

One example of chemoprophylaxis is antimalarial medication. Antimalarials have the potential for eliminating malaria from populations at risk. This has been achieved in some military groups living in endemic areas by establishing an enforced ritual and by applying sanctions against infected individuals. Soldiers are paraded daily or weekly (depending on the prophylactic used), and antimalarial tablets are ingested under supervision. In some units a check is made to ensure that the tablets have actually been swallowed. The names of participants are recorded. Disciplinary action may be taken against infected soldiers, their unit leaders, or higher commanders. The degree of departure from this ritual is accompanied by a corresponding degree of departure from malaria control. The control of malaria by chemoprophylaxis in civilian communities has never been documented.

Chemoprophylaxis is applicable to all those venereal diseases for which effective safe therapy exists. There is no reason to assume that use-effectiveness will be any greater than in other diseases for which chemoprophylaxis has been used. Antibiotic medication is associated with another serious hazard—the development of resistance. It has been demonstrated that minocycline, although given in doses sufficiently large to produce side-effects, is not uniformly effective in preventing gonorrhea. The failure rate was directly proportional to the resistance of the organisms, reaching 100 percent in the most resistant.[4] The net effect of prophylaxis with minocycline is to select resistant organisms for survival. This same process may occur for many other organisms concurrently inhabiting the host. For this reason, chemoprophylaxis with tetracycline is undesirable. Ampicillin or amoxycillin may be more effective prophylactics, but problems of improper usage or antibiotic resistance may still occur.

Immunoprophylaxis is most applicable to those diseases which themselves confer considerable and preferably lifelong immunity, are difficult to diagnose or treat, and have serious sequelae. Diseases meeting these criteria are mostly of viral etiology, but this technique is also valuable for some life-threatening bacterial infections, *e.g.*, diphtheria, tetanus. Polio provides the sole illustration of the success of immunoprophylaxis by its most rigid definition. Following the introduction of vaccines, the voluntary response exceeded all expectations, and this disease was virtually eliminated from the United States between 1960 and 1970. Possibly the crippling impact on infected children had an emotional appeal lacking for other disease-control programs. Even this appeal is not universal, however, and individuals in many underdeveloped countries have been far less receptive to voluntary polio immunization.

Many other diseases have been well controlled by immunization when some degree of persuasion has been exerted. Sanctions by the World Health Organization have virtually eliminated smallpox, plague, and yellow fever as a disease problem for soldiers and other international travelers. Sanctions by education authorities in many countries have ensured the impact of campaigns against diptheria, tetanus, and measles. In view of the poor voluntary acceptance of immunoprophylaxis for still other, more socially acceptable diseases, it seems unrealistic to expect significant utilization of venereal disease vaccines. Aside from this consideration, there are serious technical barriers to achieving control with these methods. Although yaws infection has protected many primitive communities from venereal syphilis, artificial induction of protection has proven more difficult. In view of the limited protection afforded by clinical disease, the bacterial venereal diseases are unlikely to yield to immunoprophylaxis. Since condyloma acuminatum and molluscum contagiosum are too benign to warrant the expenditure of valuable resources, genital herpes simplex and cytomegalovirus (CMV) infections should be the focus of vaccine research. The limited protection afforded by antibodies against these conditions, however, is a poor omen for the achievement of this goal.

Mass treatment. Mass treatment has been used successfully to eradicate yaws. In view of the close relationship of yaws to syphilis, it is worth considering this program in some detail. Hackett and Guthe[5] outlined the seven principles on which yaws eradication is based. All work at all stages of the campaign, including consolidation and post-campaign activities, should be planned from the outset and adequate budgetary provision made for each activity. At the time of the initial treatment, the *entire* population should be surveyed. Treatment with a long-acting penicillin preparation (PAM meeting minimum WHO requirements, or the equivalent) must be given to all persons with active yaws and to all latent cases and contacts. Periodic resurveys are essential. Data from these resurveys should be accompanied by the data of the initial treatment survey of the same population group. The expansion of the campaign should be regular and uniform so that an ever-enlarging compact area of control is formed. The reintroduction of infection by patients coming from untreated areas will then be minimal. Post-campaign activities should be planned at the outset of the campaign. If the necessary facilities for such work are not already present, simplified resurveys must continue until they have been created. Evaluation of the campaign should be made at regular intervals to ensure that the purpose of the campaign, as laid down in the plan of operations, is being achieved or to indicate modification of the plans or activities. In essence, the objective of the program is 100 percent coverage of the population at risk by house-to-house visit or assembly at a convenient site. Serology is initially performed to determine the prevalence of the disease but is not repeated. Where the prevalence exceeds 10 percent, the entire population is treated by a full dose to clinical cases and a half dose to others.

The same principles have been used for the eradication of smallpox, except that in the absence of effective therapy vaccination was used to disrupt transmission. It is important to recognize that in these campaigns, vaccination was not used in its conventional role, *i.e.*, it was not accepted voluntarily prior to risk of exposure. The role of compulsion in both yaws and smallpox control programs should be appreciated.

> Eradication schemes inevitably seem to come into conflict with human rights. So long as they depend upon compulsory immunization, mass chemotherapy, the taking of specimens of blood, urine, etc. for diagnostic purposes, the entry into homes for purposes of applying residual insecticidal sprays and for inspection purposes, the restriction of movement of personnel, etc., it will be essential that suitable enforceable legislation be adopted. Education of the public will be extremely important but it must be recognized that some violation of human rights and privileges will occur, that this is very unpopular and that the recalcitrant individual may have to be subjected to a forceful persuasion.[6]

Eradication of venereal disease in China is largely attributable to a similar policy of sacrificing the rights of individual expression and choice for the good of the community. It is unlikely, however, that such an approach is practicable in any democratic nation. The repetitive enforcement required and the almost prohibitive expense of such a policy make this approach unacceptable in these populations. If penicillin is used, a few (approximately 1/100,000 treated) noninfected individuals would die from anaphylaxis as a result of mass treatment. This is rarely a problem in primitive communities where previous exposure to penicillin is uncommon.

Screening. Although screening has been widely used in public health, it has rarely been applied to the control of infectious disease. Its major impact has been on serious, low-incidence diseases for which therapy of the established or advanced illness is suboptimal. Treatment of these conditions may be complex and of extended duration. Screening tests for these conditions should be simple, sensitive, and specific. They must be reliable, *i.e.,* provide consistant results on repetition. They must also provide a high degree of validity, that is, give a true measure of the condition being tested. The screening test must be cheap and simple, because the yield obtained is usually very low. Although sensitivity is important, its main impact is on the yield or cost-effectiveness of the program. Missed (false-negative) cases merely add to the prevalence of established disease in the community but do not disseminate disease.

Specificity is very important because of the cost, inconvenience, or side-effects of therapy. Treatment of individuals without the disease must be avoided, for the treatment may be complex, expensive, and lifelong. Consequently false-positives must be minimized. X-ray screening for tuberculosis shares some of the features of classical screening. Although this screening has been a prominent feature of programs in many countries, its impact on controlling the disease is unknown. It is essential to appreciate the differences between this type of screening and that for acute, highly contagious infections. For the latter, treatment of the established illness is often simple, safe, and cheap. Specificity is less important, for treatment of a small proportion of uninfected individuals is associated with negligible morbidity or inconvenience. Sensitivity is extremely important, however, since missed cases not only decrease the yield of screening but result in further dissemination of the disease. For this reason, the duration of the screening process is important in these diseases, because the disease will only be controlled if cases are removed more quickly than they can be generated.

Gonorrhea screening demonstrates a further diversion from classical screening. It is both relatively complicated and costly. Due to this complexity and to the need to disrupt transmission of the disease by treating a large number of infected individuals quickly, this type of screening will only be an economically effective control measure if the yield is high. In principle, indiscriminate screening is therefore an inappropriate approach to control of highly infectious diseases, particularly those with a short incubation period.

Control of venereal diseases. Epidemiologic measures for controlling venereal disease have never been fully evaluated. Even advocates of casefinding rarely support this technique for all the venereal diseases. A review of the control measures effective against other diseases indicates that individual diagnosis prior to treatment for all infected individuals is inappropriate. A community approach which inevitably involves treating some uninfected individuals is essential. At the other extreme, compulsory, repeated mass treatment is not feasible in modern democratic societies. Because of this and the limited resources available, a cost-benefit consideration must be applied to all programs. Selective mechanisms must be established to ensure that both the number of treated, uninfected individuals and number of untreated, infected individuals are minimized.

For gonorrhea, the most promising techniques currently available are selective screening and epidemiologic treatment. The cost-benefit of screening depends on the yield of positive cases, the effort involved in the process, the seriousness of the sequelae prevented, and the cost of screening. For example, screening for syphilis during pregnancy may be justified if only one case per 10,000 is detected. A similar yield in the total population makes this procedure uneconomic. Screening at medical facilities where genital examinations are routinely performed is more economical than in situations where individuals congregate for the specific purpose of screening. Where a gonorrhea yield of 5 percent or less may be uneconomic in the latter situation, it may be justified in the former.

The proportion of detected cases in those screened determines the economy of the procedure, but the control effectiveness of this technique is related to the proportion of infected individuals not screened and the duration of the screening process. It is essential that the target group is carefully delineated, not only to ensure high yield from those screened but also to minimize the number of infected individuals who escape the screen.

Epidemiologic treatment refers to antibiotic administration when a diagnosis is considered likely on epidemiologic grounds prior to proof of infection by laboratory methods. It follows that only the full therapeutic dose of the antibiotic is used. The decision to treat should be determined by the following factors: the risk of infection, the seriousness of the disease, the difficulties in diagnosis, the efficacy of treatment, the side-effects of treatment, the likelihood of further disease dissemination, and the likelihood of patient followup. Treatment of gonorrhea on the basis of laboratory diagnosis is recommended for asymptomatic males with a negative Gram smear if the physician is virtually certain of patient followup and if there is negligible chance of transmission in the surveillance period. In other situations, epidemiologic treatment should be considered. This applies to all sexual contacts of a proven case of gonococcal infection. Epidemiologic treatment can be viewed as selective mass treatment. Selected groups of patients with a high risk of infection are identified by various parameters and treated before confirmation of their infection status. This reduces infection in three ways: 1) it ensures treatment for those who could not be located or would not return when notified of positive test results. 2) Those who do return may continue to transmit the infection between time of testing and treatment. 3) It is the most practicable method by which those infected women with false-negative endocervical cultures will receive treatment. Although this procedure results in treating many uninfected individuals, it increases the chance of disrupting transmission, a condition essential for control of the disease.

Neither epidemiologic treatment nor selective screening can be applied on a rational basis without a sound knowledge of the epidemiology of disease in any particular environment (as listed in Figures 12-5, 12-6, and 12-7). Without this knowledge, these techniques are unlikely to be effective.

Attitudes to Disease and Health Services

Although it is easier to develop new methods of control than it is to change human behavior, increased understanding of the factors influencing public response will enable better utilization of the scientific control aids now available. Failure to make effective contact with problem groups results primarily from assumptions that individuals in these groups behave in an essentially rational manner and that they have values similar to those of medical authorities or other middle-class members of society. Unless these assumptions are discarded, the dismal record of venereal disease control will be perpetuated. Persons in these problem groups have values differing widely from those of medical authorities nor do they view venereal disease as a serious illness. Long-term health risks provide less motivation to seek health care than immediate discomfort or inconvenience. The low reported incidence of nongonococcal urethritis in some communities is most commonly a result of this attitude. This condition, which often resolves spontaneously, causes minimal discomfort and is readily ignored by the apathetic patient. The same phenomenon commonly occurs with syphilis, which may produce a painless ulcer that heals spontaneously in a few weeks. Some patients even ignore gonorrhea until the offensive odor or the continual soiling of clothing by urethral discharge proves intolerable. In all these situations, medical care is finally sought, not for its intrinsic benefit, but because it is the lesser of two inconveniences.

This apathy is not merely a result of ignorance of the consequences of venereal disease; it results from special attitudes or beliefs found in high-risk groups. Many individuals fail to use a condom either because they find it inconvenient or because they believe that they are not susceptible to venereal disease. It is one of those distasteful diseases acquired only by people in a lower socioeconomic class. For similar reasons, some individuals refuse to participate in screening programs or to accept epidemiologic treatment—although many may have venereal disease. Present evidence suggests that the same problems would be encountered in gaining acceptance of immunization if vaccines for the venereal diseases were developed.

Many individuals are largely motivated to seek health care for non-health related reasons. Peer values or pressures are the most potent motivators, but sanctions imposed by employers or public administration are solely responsible for bringing some individuals to medical attention. As mentioned above, forceful persuasion has made a major contribution to immunization campaigns in most environments.

From this understanding of patient motivation, public participation in control can be maximized by adopting a number of policies. First of all, health care must be made convenient for potential patients. Clinics should be located in the areas where most patients live or work. Large shopping complexes in high-risk areas are obvious clinic sites, but if care must be delivered to a wide area, mobile clinics may be useful for some services. When it is more convenient to accept medical care than deliberately to avoid it, greater utilization can be anticipated.

The demands on public response should be minimized. Complex techniques or theoretical campaigns may be counterproductive if they discourage repeated use. The venereal disease patient or suspect favors a brief convenient clinic visit which is psychologically and physically as atraumatic as possible. Unnecessary or insensitive interrogation by an interviewer may locate a few extra contacts, but it may also eliminate any possibility of cooperation with the whole social group. Treatment should be as simple and untraumatic as possible, and unnecessary surveillance must be avoided. A patient who willingly keeps one or two surveillance appointments may be discouraged from any participation if four or five further visits are suggested. Failure to adopt these principles may alienate large social groups, such as homosexuals or teenagers, from the clinic system.

It is important that health-care users accept and identify with health-care personnel. Consequently, race, age, and socioeconomic class are important considerations when employing staff. In selection, these factors may take precedence over formal qualifications or training. Currently, one of the greatest defects in many clinics is the preponderance of older, disinterested physicians and antisocial supporting staff. These personnel understand no one and antagonize everyone.

Existing social organizations should be mobilized to participate in control campaigns. In the past, unfortunately, the choice of supporting organizations such as the church and police has been glaringly inappropriate. The inevitable result of their participation has been to alienate those very groups—prostitutes, homosexuals, the highly promiscuous, and racial minority groups—whose cooperation is essential. Assistance should be sought instead directly from those target groups who should be represented in control campaigns and health-delivery services.

Casefinding

Social workers were first used for VD work in Europe early in the twentieth century. Extensions of these early techniques are now widely used in venereal disease control programs. The contribution of contact tracing was demonstrated by an early study in 1947 in Arkansas where 201 patients named 655 sex contacts, of whom 167 were found to have previously undiagnosed syphilis.[7]

Briefly, contact tracing consists of a contact interview with the infected patient to establish contacts or those who were sex partners during the critical time period of infectivity. The interview is followed by a contact investigation to locate and bring in these contacts for examination and treatment if it is required. This method can be expanded by examining cluster suspects, persons named by the patient who were not sex partners during the critical period, and cluster associates, individuals who have a social relationship with the patient. The most sophisticated ideal of tracing is speed zone epidemiology whereby an attempt is made to intercept gonococcal infection within its incubation period.

Cluster suspects are commonly mentioned by the patient because they have lesions similar to those of the patient, because they have intimate contact with friends or partners of the patient, or because they are sexual partners or friends of previously infected patients. Approximately 3 percent of cluster associates may have VD.[8]

In one study, 204 cases of primary and secondary syphilis yielded 387 contacts, of whom 343 (88.7 percent) were examined. Of these contacts, 258 (75.3 percent) had syphilis, which was infectious in 213 (62 percent).[8] Not all results are so impressive, however. More commonly, a much smaller proportion of contacts can be traced, and these yield a lower return of patients. Wigfield[9] summarized the results from the Tyneside scheme that covers an area in England with a current population of 1.5 million. By 1970, 19,721 male and female contacts had been recorded, but there was sufficient information to locate only 9,590 (48.5 percent). Of these, 4,030 (42 percent) had VD. In a London clinic, 119 men named 145 recent sexual partners, of whom only 48 percent could be traced.[10] In a Newcastle study,[11] only 58 percent of 2855 patients gave reliable information enabling 1560 contacts to be examined. The examinations disclosed that 70 percent had VD. Lamb[12] had even less success in locating contacts (12.1 percent of syphilis contacts and 19.7 percent of the gonorrhea contacts), although a high infection rate (77 percent for syphilis and 82.5 percent for gonorrhea) was found among those who were located.

In one area, Blount[13] reported voluntary attendance of 95 percent of male patients but only 36 percent of females. Of the male contacts named by female patients, 61 percent had symptomatic gonorrhea at the time of investigation. Contact tracing apparently provides its greatest contribution in bringing to treatment the often asymptomatic female contacts of male patients; however, contact tracing may be the simplest method of detecting asymptomatic male infection. The asymptomatic male contacts of symptomatic females should therefore provide a significant yield of gonococcal infections, although they may be only a small proportion of the total number of contact cases. The goal of contact tracing is to bring to treatment the asymptomatic contacts of infected patients, regardless of their sex.

Contact tracing is expensive and time consuming, and it has been suggested that one full-time contact tracer and supporting staff is required for every eight new registrations per day.[9] Due to these costs, tracing visits may be replaced by telephone calls, writing, or patient assistance.

A tracing team consists of the clinician, interviewer/investigator, and the supporting staff. Success is facilitated by a relaxed atmosphere and mutual respect both between team members and with the patients with whom they work.

It is clearly impracticable to attempt to trace all sexual contacts of all patients. Selection should be guided by the severity of the disease and the likelihood that the infected contact will not otherwise seek treatment. Consequently, asymptomatic contacts of patients with gonorrhea and all syphilis contacts usually receive priority.

The simplest form of tracing merely involves asking the patient to refer his or her contacts for treatment. With greater sophistication and available resources, contact interviewers and contact investigators are employed. Although preferred in these roles, social workers are not always available and other paramedical workers must be employed. It should be emphasized that these tasks are highly specialized and require skilled personnel of high integrity. Thorough screening is essential to ensure that only those with adequate training, suitable attitudes, and acceptable personalities are employed in these roles.

Although there is inevitably some overlap in the tasks of the tracing team, and while all are involved in interviewing, repetition should be minimized and the role of each member clearly delineated. Preferably the clinician assesses the period of infectivity and provides the interviewer with a definite period within which to elicit information about contacts and associates. The interviewer therefore need not discuss clinical or epidemiologic aspects of venereal disease with the patient, other than in the most elementary fashion required for conducting a fluent conversation with the patient. All detailed inquiry about such topics as possible means of transmission, infectivity, and clinical sequelae should be referred to the clinician. Although this policy is contrary to widespread practice there are three related reasons favoring its implementation. To answer the technical questions asked by patients often requires a sophisticated knowledge of venereal infection not always possessed by social workers. A clear distinction must always be made between possible and probable modes of transmission. The patient should be discouraged from indulgence in theoretical hypotheses that are fruitless and unnecessarily aggravate the social impact of infection. When more than one individual provides technical information, the patient becomes confused and possibly agitated should this information differ from one source to another. Often the clinician must investigate clinical and epidemiologic problems in some depth to provide efficient management. Any doubts or uncertainty expressed by the patient are very relevant in assessing the emotional or neurotic sequelae of infection and thus its management.

Clearly, the sex partners of infected patients constitute an important high-prevalence reservoir of infection. Although of some value for syphilis, the conventional syphilis contact interview procedure is too time consuming, expensive, and cumbersome to cope with an epidemic of a disease with a very short incubation period. Other methods of bringing large numbers of contacts to treatment rapidly must be investigated. Methods that use the patient as an intermediary are probably the most promising. In any case, it is essential for the physician to emphasize to all patients the importance, for their own health as well as for disease control, of having their sex partners receive early treatment. The ideal situation, which can be stressed in education programs, would be for patients and their sex partners initially to visit the medical facility together.

Assessing Venereal Disease Incidence

Because of limitations of staff, facilities, or finance, most control programs will be unable to cope with the requirements of the control phase, much less progress beyond this stage. A prerequisite for a genuine effort to control VD is accurate assessment of the incidence of infection. In most communities the reported incidence of infection represents only a small proportion of the actual incidence. In developed communities where reporting is compulsory, this is largely due to apathy and deception, but the most common worldwide reason for this discrepancy is poor communication. Many infected individuals do not have access to medical care, while others are seen by attendants who are unable to formulate an accurate diagnosis. Even where diagnosis is made, the mechanism for collecting and collating data is often poorly developed or nonexistent.

With the development of a control program, the reported incidence of infection may rise dramatically as these deficiencies are corrected (Figure 12-10). Although incidence will stabilize when all cases are reported, a steady rate may indicate merely a new base line of inefficiency, and a falling rate may suggest a breakdown in program application. In the attack phase, the incidence falls to a maintenance level characterized by its stability over a long period rather than by any actual incidence level. Rising or fluctuating levels within this phase indicate that control has been lost.

Compulsory notification of venereal disease by practicing doctors has proven inadequate in assessing the incidence of infection. It is doubtful whether this policy serves any useful purpose. By contrast, compulsory notification by pathology laboratories of all venereal disease tests performed provides a reliable method of monitoring infection in the community, although it will fail to disclose infections treated by doctors who do not use laboratory diagnostic aids.

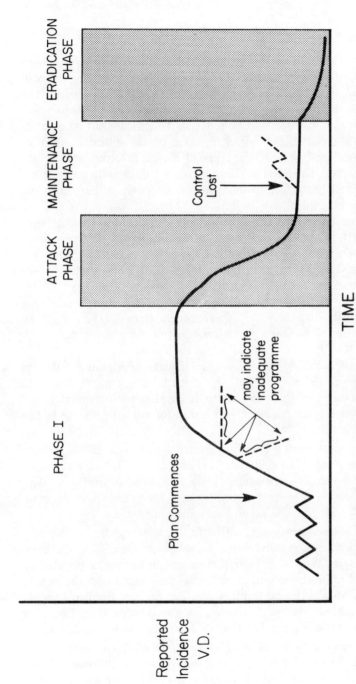

FIGURE 12-10 VARIATION OF REPORTED INCIDENCE OF VD RELATED TO PHASE OF VD CONTROL

Attack Phase

The attack phase can be instituted when a control plan has been fully developed and sufficient resources are available to implement policies that follow from the accumulated epidemiologic knowledge. The initial step in this phase involves allocating a maintenance level to which venereal disease incidence is to be reduced. This should not be an arbitrary or idealistic level but one determined by the intrinsic nature of the sociological environment, the types of disease involved, and the resources available. This level is thus not related to the efficiency of the controlling staff but rather to those factors over which the controlling program has no control.

Prerequisites for the attack phase include adequate clinical facilities and staff to provide acceptable management for all those being tested or treated. There is no substitute for this requirement. Controllers should never attempt to compensate for clinical inadequacies by increased expenditure on other components of the control program. Bringing contacts or suspects to a clinic serves no useful purpose unless they can be correctly diagnosed and appropriately treated. There must be prior allocation of sufficient funds for the full duration of the attack phase as well as funds to provide adequate maintenance.

A precise knowledge of the geographic and sociological distribution of the disease in the community is basic to the attack phase. Certainly precise knowledge of that part of the infected community that is not utilizing health services together with a plan for reducing disease in this group is mandatory.

Finally, there must be an established liaison with all the private physicians and medical facilities in the control area and a mechanism for maintaining their cooperation during the future control campaign. With this, there must be mechanisms for monitoring disease in the community and evaluating the control measures instituted.

The attack program must be flexible, for the emphasis on different techniques may vary rapidly as the prevalence of disease in the community changes. With very high prevalence throughout a population, it is essential to bring the total population into contact with the health-care system. Mobile clinical facilities may be required. Emphasis should be placed on epidemiologic treatment. Diagnostic tests should be used as a guide to prevalence rather than as an indication for treatment.

As prevalence falls and disease is eliminated from some groups, screening of the remaining high-prevalence pockets of infection should be undertaken. The correlation of screening yield with epidemiologic data provides the criteria for epidemiologic treatment. If the program is effective, these correlations and consequently the criteria for treatment may change rapidly. Constant monitoring of screening yields and periodic adjustment of criteria for epidemiologic treatment is consequently essential.

With low prevalence of infection in certain well-defined groups, interviewing techniques become feasible. Indeed, at this stage of control, interviews are the most economical means of bringing infected persons to treatment.

Maintenance Phase

In the maintenance phase, infection is removed from the community as rapidly as it is introduced or generated. Population size, mobility, and behavioral patterns are important determinants of the actual level at which the prevalence can be maintained. These factors will also influence the resources required for stable maintenance. In some environments, the demand on resources will be almost as great as in the attack phase. In others, a great reduction is compatible with stability. Excessive reduction makes a resurgence of infection possible.

In the maintenance phase, case reporting and contact tracing are important. The number of cases is relatively small, and these tend to occur in groups so that these techniques are feasible. Epidemiologic treatment should still be used, however, and all sex partners of detected cases should be treated as soon as contacted without waiting for the results of diagnostic tests.

Eradication Phase

Eradication should be attemped only in those environments where it is possible, through effective monitoring, to maintain the community virtually free of infection. In large cosmopolitan mobile communities, eradication is not only difficult or impossible, but would serve no useful purpose if established. Venereal disease would be continually reintroduced, and a brief minor lapse in the control program would enable the rapid restoration of a high infection prevalence.

Future Prospects of Venereal Disease Control

A clear distinction should be drawn between extrinsic problems of control—such as prejudice, apathy, and inadequate allocation of resources—and intrinsic problems that relate to the nature of the diseases and the behavioral characteristics of the individuals who acquire them. Due to a long incubation period, effective therapy, and satisfactory serologic diagnostic aids, the main barriers to syphilis control are extrinsic.

Although extrinsic factors greatly hinder control of the contagious urethrites, their control is currently precluded by intrinsic factors—a short incubation period, a high prevalence of asymptomatic infection, and the absence of a suitable serologic screening test. There is currently no means to counter the spread of gonorrhea among highly mobile promiscuous individuals. Determining the causative organisms of nongonococcal urethritis, which probably differ considerably from one environment to another, would greatly alleviate the morbidity from anxiety and the unnecessary treatment which results from the absence of unambiguous diagnostic criteria of infection and cure.

Of considerable importance in predicting future control is the fact that venereal disease presents a moving target. It is unrealistic to consider that solution of current problems will eliminate the impact of these diseases. New problems are constantly appearing, both from the disclosure of previously unrecognized phenomena and from real changes in venereal disease epidemiology. The increasing resistance of the gonococcus to penicillin has been a subject of much research in the past decade. An increasing awareness of asymptomatic infection in the male and asymptomatic extragenital gonococcal infection with apparent increased resistance to treatment must provoke considerable concern among many venereologists.

In the unlikely event that the infective conditions seen at venereal disease clinics are reduced to negligible incidence in the near future, the venereologist will still be confronted by difficult problems in many areas of psychosocial maladjustment. This field of sexual adjustment has been virtually neglected by the community and the medical profession alike. Despite the severe social morbidity from this problem and an abundance of pseudoexperts, effective techniques have not been devised for consistently influencing human behavior so that harmful sequelae to sexual behavior are minimized. For these reasons, venereology is likely to remain one of the most interesting and challenging fields of medicine in the future.

Notes

Foreword

1. Lucas JB, Gonorrhea, in Top, FH and Wehrle, PF, eds: Communicable and infectious diseases, 7th ed, CV Mosby, St Louis, 1972, 277

Chapter One—Introduction

1. Parkinson CN: Parkinson's law, Houghton Mifflin, Boston 1957
2. Fleming WL, Brown WJ, Donohue R, Branigan PW: National survey of venereal disease treated by physicians in 1968, JAMA, 211: 1827, 1970
3. Curtis AC: The reported and actual morbidity of syphilis and gonorrhea, Arch Environ Health, 13: 381, 1966
4. World Health Organization: Control of gonococcal infections, WHO Chron 18: 14, 1964
5. Willcox RR: A worldwide view of venereal disease, Br J Vener Dis, 48: 163, 1972
6. Kackler J, Brolnitsky O, Orbach H: Preliminary report on a mass program for detection of gonorrhea, Public Health Rep, 85: 681, 1970
7. Catterall RD, Morton RS: Crisis in venereology, Br Med J 3: 699, 1970
8. Greenberg JH: Venereal disease in the armed forces, Med Clin North Amer 56: 1087, 1972

9. Ratcliffe TA: Psychiatric and allied aspects of the problem of venereal disease in the army: with particular reference to S.E.A.C., J R Army Med Cps 89: 122, 1947

10. Hinrichsen J: Venereal disease in the major armies and navies of the world, Am J Syph Gonor Vener Dis, 28: 736, 1944

11. King A: Failure to control venereal disease, Br Med J 1: 451, 1970

12. Willcox RR: Fifty years since the conception of an organisational VD service in Great Britain, Br J Vener Dis 43: 1, 1967

13. Dwyer JM: Notes on male venereology, S Austral Clin 3: 216, 1968

14. Glass LH: An analysis of some characteristics of males with gonorrhea, Br J Vener Dis 43: 128, 1967

Chapter Two—Sex Education for Health Professionals

1. Wabrek AJ, Feldman PM: Human aspects of medical sexuality, Obstet Gynecol 39: 805, 1972

2. Mace DR, Bannermann RHO, Burton J: The teaching of human sexuality in schools for health professionals, WHO Public Health Pap 57, Geneva, Switzerland,

Chapter Three—Normal and Abnormal Sexual Behavior

1. Davis K: Sexual behavior, in Merton RK, Nisbet R: Contemporary social problems, 3rd ed, Harcourt Brace Jovanovich, New York, 1971

2. Stokes RE: Sexual deviation and venereal disease, Public Health Rep 997: 444, 1964

3. Ellis A: Coitus, in Encyclopedia of sexual behavior, Corsano, London, 1961

4. Morgenthau JE, Sokoloff NJ: The sexual revolution: myth or fact? Pediatr Clin North Amer, 19: 779, 1972

5. Biegel AC: Abstinence, in Ellis A, Abarbanel, A., Encyclopedia of sexual behavior 41, Corsano, London, 1961

6. Terman LM: Psychological factors in marital happiness, McGraw-Hill, New York, 1938

7. Bell RR: Premarital sex in a changing society, Prentice Hall, Englewood Cliffs, N.J., 1966

8. McCance C, Hall DJ: Sexual behavior and contraceptive practice of female undergraduates at Aberdeen University, Br Med J 2: 694, 1972

9. Hart G: The impact of prostitution on Australian troops at war, unpubl doctoral thesis, U Adelaide, South Australia, 1974

10. Dearborn LW: Auto-eroticism, in Encyclopedia of sexual behavior op cit, 1961

11. Kinsey AC, Pomeroy WB, Martin CE: Sexual behavior in the human male, 1st ed, WB Saunders, London, 1948

12. Hohmann LB, Schaffner B: The sex lives of unmarried men, Am J Sociol, 52: 501, 1947

13. Broderick CB, Bernard J: The individual, sex and society, Johns Hopkins Press, Baltimore, 1969

14. Comfort A: The anxiety makers, Panther Books, London, 1968

15. Kinsey, Pomeroy, Martin: Sexual behavior in the human male

16. Kellogg R: Babies need fathers too, New York, 1953

17. Reiss AJ: The social integration of queers and peers, Soc Probl 9: 102, 1961

18. Allen C: A textbook of psychosocial disorders, 2nd ed, Oxford University Press, London, 1969

19. Morris D: Intimate behavior, Jonathan Cape, London, 1971

20. Ellis: Coitus

21. Hart: Impact of prostitution on Australian troops

22. Kinsey, Pomeroy, Martin: Sexual behavior in the human male

23. Saghir MT, Robins E, Walbran B: Homosexuality. II. Sexual behavior of the male homosexual, Arch Gen Psychiatry 21: 219, 1969

24. Henriques F: Modern sexuality, Panther Books, London, 1969

25. Pariser H: Asymptomatic gonorrhea, Med Clin North Am 56: 1127, 1972

26. Broderick, Bernard: The individual, sex, and society

27. Pariser H, Marino AF: Gonorrhea: frequently unrecognized reservoirs, South Med J 63: 198, 1970

28. Owen RL, Hill JL: Rectal and pharyngeal gonorrhea in homosexual men, JAMA 220: 1315, 1972

29. Pariser, Marino: Gonorrhea

30. Pariser: Asymptomatic gonorrhea

31. Pariser: Asymptomatic gonorrhea

Chapter Four—Prevention and Management of Unwanted Pregnancy

1. In this discussion, legal factors, which are highly variable from one community to another, are not considered. Statutory restrictions in some areas will preclude application of the medicosocial principles advocated.

2. World Health Organization: Advances in Fertility Control, WHO Chron 26: 12, 1972

3. Committee of the Institute of Medicine: Legalized abortion and the public health, Nat Acad Sci, Washington, 1975

Chapter Five—Promiscuity and Prostitution

1. Wittkower ED: The psychological aspects of venereal disease, Br J Vener Dis 24: 59, 1948
2. Scheinfeld A: Women and men, Chatto Windus, London, 1947
3. Clinard MB: The sociology of deviant behavior, Holt Rinehart Winston, New York, 1963
4. Willcox RR: Prostitution and venereal disease, Antiseptic, 60: 1, 1963
5. Scheinfeld: Women and men
6. Greenwald H. The call girl, Holt and Co, New York, 1958
7. Davis K: Sexual behavior, in Merton RK, Nisbet R: Contemporary social problems, 3rd ed, Harcourt Brace Jovanovich, New York, 1971
8. Oliven JF: Sexual hygiene and pathology, Lippincott, Philadelphia, 1965
9. Henriques F: Modern sexuality, Panther, London, 1969
10. Henriques F: Stews and strumpets, 1st ed, MacGibbon and Kee, London, 1961
11. Willcox: Prostitution and venereal disease
12. Bettley PR: The medical conduct of a brothel, Br J Vener Dis 25: 56, 1949
13. Lentino W: Medical evaluation of a system of legalised prostitution, JAMA, 158: 20, 1955
14. Major RH: War and disease, Hutchinsons, Melbourne, 1944
15. Dudley S: The prevention of venereal disease in the Royal Navy, J R Nav Med Serv 53: 39, 1967
16. Bullough VL: History of prostitution in the United States, Med Aspects Human Sex, 4: 64, 1970
17. Lees R. Venereal disease in the armed forces overseas, Br J Vener Dis 22: 149, 1946
18. Henriques: Stews and strumpets
19. Greenberg JH: Venereal disease in the armed forces, Med Clin North Am 56: 1087, 1972
20. Lees: Venereal disease in the armed forces overseas
21. Curtis FR: Venereal disease in the British occupied zone of Germany, Br J Vener Dis 23: 20, 1947
22. Henriques F: The immoral tradition, Panther, London, 1966

23. Hinrichsen J: Venereal disease in the major armies and navies of the world, J Syph Gonor Vener Dis 28: 736, 1944

24. Willcox: Prostitution and venereal disease

25. Willcox RR: Factors leading to a failure of control of gonorrhea, Br J Prev Soc Med, 16: 113, 1962

26. Curtis: Venereal disease in the British occupied zone

27. Greenberg: Venereal disease in the British occupied zone

28. Lees: Venereal disease in the armed forces overseas

29. Henriques: The immoral tradition

30. Henriques: Modern sexuality

31. Wren BG: Gonorrhea among prostitutes, Med J Aust 1: 847, 1967

32. Adler P: A house is not a home, Harborough, London, 1954

33. Mancini J: Body painting: the youngest profession, in Nobile P: The new eroticism, 1st ed, Random House, New York, 1970

34. Adler: A house is not a home

35. Hijmans A: Prostitution, promiscuity and prophylaxis, Rotterdam Port Demonstration Center 1953–1954, WHO Publ, 1956

36. Schwartz O: The psychology of sex, Penguin, Middlesex, 1949

37. Scheinfeld: Women and men

38. Adler: A house is not a home

39. Jackman NR, O'Toole R, Geis G: The self image of the prostitute, Sociol Q 4: 150, 1963

40. Henriques: Modern sexuality

41. Davis KO: The sociology of prostitution, Am Sociol Rev 2: 746, 1937

42. Henriques: Modern sexuality

43. Greenwald: The call girl

44. Henriques: Modern sexuality

45. Henriques: Modern sexuality

46. Adler: A house is not a home

47. Esselstyn TC: Prostitution in the United States, Am Acad Pol Soc Sci 376: 123, 1968

48. Henriques: Modern sexuality

49. Oller LZ, Wood T: Factors influencing the incidence of gonorrhea and non-gonococcal urethritis in men in an industrial city, Br J Vener Dis 46: 96, 1970

50. Clinard: The sociology of deviant behavior

51. Sanger WW: The history of prostitution, 2nd ed, Medical Publishing, New York, 1919

52. Sieff B: Venereal disease in South Africa. Sociological aspects, Med Proc 12: 224, 1966

53. Henriques: Modern sexuality

54. Lees: Venereal disease in the armed forces overseas

55. Henriques: Modern sexuality

56. Graham RS: Venereal disease conditions in the Far East, Am J Syph 36: 433, 1952

57. Henriques: Stews and strumpets

58. Henriques: Modern sexuality

59. Henriques: The immoral tradition

60. Social background of venereal disease, Tyneside experimental scheme in venereal disease control. October 1943 to March 1944, Br J Vener Dis 21: 26.

61. Idsoe O, Guthe T: The rise and fall of the treponematoses. I. Ecological aspects and international trends in venereal syphilis, Br J Vener Dis 43: 227, 1967 Johns HM: The social aspects of the venereal diseases. 3. Contact tracing, Br J Vener Dis 21: 17, 1945

62. Henriques: Modern sexuality

63. Mancini: Body painting

64. Davis: Sexual behavior

65. Henriques: Modern sexuality

66. Clinard: The sociology of deviant behavior

67. Bryan JH: Apprenticeship in prostitution, Soc Probl 12: 287, 1965

68. Henriques: Modern sexuality

69. Adler: A house is not a home

70. Henriques: Stews and strumpets

71. Hijmans: Prostitution, promiscuity and prophylaxis

72: Davis: Sexual behavior

73: Daxis: Sexual behavior

74. Prebble EE: Venereal disease in India, Br J Vener Dis 22: 55, 1956 Walker AS: Clinical problems of war, Halstead Press, Sydney, 1952 Shah JM: Sex life in India and Pakistan, in Ellis A, Abarbanel A., Encyclopedia of sexual behavior, 528 Corsano, London, 1961

75. Stuart J: V.D. contacts of merchant seamen, Rotterdam Port Demonstration Center 1953–1954. WHO Publ, 1956

76. Ross AOF: The different aspects of maritime venereal-disease control, Rotterdam Port Demonstration Center 1953–1954, WHO Publi, 1956

77. Platts WM: Venereal disease in New Zealand, Br J Vener Dis 45: 61, 1969

Chapter Six—Homosexuality and Homosexual Behavior

1. Reiss AJ: The social integration of queers and peers, Soc Probl 9: 102, 1961
2. Ford CS, Beach FA: Patterns of sexual behavior, Methuen, London, 1965
3. Kinsey AC, Pomeroy WB, Martin CE: Sexual behavior in the human male, WB Saunders, London, 1948
4. Bieber I: Conclusions of homosexuality: a psychoanalytical study of male homosexuals, in McCaffrey JA, The homosexual dialectic, Prentice Hall, Englewood Cliffs, N.J., 1972
5. West DJ: Homosexuality, Duckworth Co, London, 1968
6. Saghir MI, Robins E, Walbran B: Homosexuality. II. Sexual behavior in the male homosexual, Arch Gen Psychiatry 21: 219, 1969
7. Williams CJ, Weinberg MS: The military. Its processing of accused homosexuals. Am Behav Sci 14: 203, 1970
8. Henriques F: Modern sexuality, 57, Panther, London, 1969
9. Hohmann LB, Schaffner B: The sex lives of unmarried men, Am J Sociol 52: 501, 1947
10. Tarr JF, Lugar RR: Early infectious syphilis: male homosexual relations as a mode of spread, Calif Med 93: 35, 1960 Trice ER, Clark FA: Transmission of venereal diseases through homosexual practices, South Med J 54: 76, 1961

Chapter Seven—The Venereal Diseases

1. King A, Nicol C: Venereal diseases, 2nd ed, Bailliere Tindall Cassell, London, 1969
2. Willcox RR: A textbook of venereal diseases and treponematoses, 2nd ed, Heinemann, London, 1964
3. Schofield CBS: Sexually transmitted diseases, Churchill Livingstone, Edinburgh, 1972
4. Report of Chief Medical Officer for 1972: sexually transmitted diseases, Br J Vener Dis 50: 57, 1975
5. Mayou R: Psychological morbidity in a clinic for sexually transmitted disease, Br J Vener Dis 51; 57, 1975
6. McCormack WM: Management of sexually transmissible infections during pregnancy, Clin Obstet Gynecol 18: 57, 1975
7. Hart G, Rein M: Gonococcal infection, in Top FH, Wehrle PF, eds, Communicable and infectious diseases, 8th ed, Mosby, St Louis, 1976

8. Hart G: Penicillin resistance of gonococci in South Vietnam, Med J Aust 2: 638, 1973

9. McChesney JA et al: Acute urethritis in male college students, JAMA 226: 37, 1973

10. Jacobs NF, Kraus JS: Gonococcal and nongonococcal urethritis in men, Ann Intern Med 82: 7, 1975

11. Schroeter AL, Lucas JB: Gonorrhea—diagnosis and treatment, Obstet Gynec 39: 274, 1972

12. Wiesner PJ: Diagnostic problems in gonorrhea, Presented at 3rd Int Vener Dis Symp, New Orleans, 1973

13. Handsfield HH et al: Asymptomatic gonorrhea in men. Diagnosis, natural course, prevalence, and significance, N Engl J Med 209: 117, 1974

14. Sutherland R, Croydon EAP, Rolinson GN: Amoxicillin: a new semisynthetic penicillin, Br Med J 3: 13, 1972

15. McCormack WM, et al: The genital mycoplasmas, N Engl J Med 228: 78, 1973

16. Richmond SJ, et al: Chlamydial infection: role of chlamydia subgroup A in nongonococcal and post gonococcal urethritis, Br J Vener Dis 48: 437, 1973

17. Handsfield HH, et al: Etiology and treatment of nongonococcal urethritis, Twelfth Interscience Conf on Antimicrobial Agents and Chemotherapy, Atlantic City, New Jersey, 1972

18. Nahmias AJ, Roizman B: Infection with herpes simplex viruses 1 and 2, N Engl J Med 289: 667, 719, 781, 1973

19. Kaufman RH, Rawls WE: Herpes genitalis and its relationship to cervical cancer, CA 24: 258, 1974

20. Jirovec O, Petro M: Trichomonas vaginalis and trichomoniasis, Adv Parasitol 6: 117, 1968

21. Syphilis: a synopsis, Public Health Rep 1660, 1968

22. Hart G: The diagnosis of syphilis, Med J Aust 2: 722, 1975

23. Weller TH: The cytomegaloviruses: Ubiquitous agents with protean clinical manifestations, N Engl J Med 285: 203, 267, 1971

24. Jordan MC, et al: Association of cervical cytomegaloviruses with venereal disease, N Engl J Med 287: 932, 1973

25. Hart G: Chancroid, Donovanosis, Lymphogranuloma Venereum, HEW Publ (CDC) 75-8302, 1975

26. Lal S, Nicholas C: Epidemiological and clinical features in 165 cases of granuloma inguinale, Br J Vener Dis 46: 461, 1970

27. Lewis JF, et al: Corynebacterium vaginale vaginitis, Am J Obstet Gynecol 112: 87, 1972

28. Akerlund M, Mardh PA: Isolation and identification of Coryne-bacterium vaginale (Haemophilis vaginalis) in women with infections of the lower genital tract. Acta Obstet Gynecol Scand 53: 85, 1974

29. Oriel JD: Natural history of genital warts, Br J Vener Dis 47: 1, 1971

30. Powell LC, Pollard M, Jinkins JL: Treatment of condylomata acuminata by autogenous vaccine, South Med J 63: 202, 1970

31. Drake TE, Maibach HI: Candida and candidiasis, Postgrad Med 53: 83, 120, 1973

Chapter Eight—Environmental and Individual Factors

1. Wittkower ED, Cowan J: Some psychological aspects of sexual promiscuity, Psychsom Med 6: 287, 1944

2. Ford CS, Beach FA: Patterns of sexual behavior, Methuen, London, 1965

3. Kinsey AC, Pomeroy WB, Martin CE: Sexual behavior in the human male, WB Saunders, London, 1948

4. Reiss IL: Premarital sexual standards in America, Free Press, Glencoe, 1960

5. Wessell MA, Pinck BD: Venereal disease anxiety, J Ment Hyg 31: 636, 1947

6. Prebble EE: Venereal disease in India, Br J Vener Dis 22: 55, 1946

7. Stouffer SA, Suchman EA, De Vinney LC, Star SA, Williams RM: The American soldier, John Wiley Sons, New York, 1965

8. Butler AG: Official history of the Australian army medical services 1914–18. Vol. III. Problems and services, Australian War Memorial, Canberra, 1943

9. Greenberg JH: Venereal disease in the armed forces, Med Clin North Am 56: 1087, 1972

10. Hinrichsen J: Venereal disease in the major armies and navies of the world, Part II, J Syph Gonor Vener Dis, 29: 80, 1945

11. Ratcliffe TA: Psychiatric and allied aspects of the problem of venereal disease in the army: with particular reference to S.E.A.C., J R Army Med. Cps 89: 122, 1947

12. Norris FK: No memory for pain, Heinemann, Melbourne, 1970

13. Ehrmann W: Premarital dating behavior, Henry Holt Co, New York, 1959

14. Gardner GE: Sex behavior of adolescents in wartime, Ann Am Acad Pol Sci 236: 60, 1944

15. Elkin H: Aggressive and erotic tendencies in army life, Am J Sociol 51: 408, 1946

16. McCallum MR: The study of the delinquent in the army, Am J Sociol 51: 479, 1946

17. Sutherland R: Some individual and social factors in venereal disease, Br J Vener Dis 26: 1, 1950

18. Brown WJ: The status of gonorrhea in the U.S.A. and current problems in its control, Bull WHO 24: 386, 1961

19. Glass LH: An analysis of some characteristics of males with gonorrhea, Br J Vener Dis 43: 128, 1967

20. Lomholt G, Berg O: Gonorrhea situation in South Greenland in the summer of 1964, Br J Vener Dis 42: 1, 1966

21. Hart G: Sexual behavior in a war environment, J Sex Res 11: 218, 1974

22. Brody MW: Men who contract venereal diseases, J Vener Dis Inform, 29: 334, 1948

23. Blair HI: The venereal disease problem in a woman's federal reformatory, Am J Syph Gonor Vener Dis 30: 165, 1946

24. Bowdoin CD: Socioeconomic factors in syphilis prevalence, Savannah, Georgia, J Vener Dis Inform, 30: 131, 1949

25. Burney LE: Control of syphilis in a southern rural area, Am J Public Health, 29: 1006, 1939

26. Willcox RR: Venereal disease in British West Africa, Br J Vener Dis 22: 63, 1946

27. Platts WM: Venereal disease in New Zealand, Br J Vener Dis 45: 61, 1969

28. Idsoe O, Kiraly K, Causse G: Venereal disease and treponematoses—the epidemiological situation and WHO's control program, WHO Chron 27: 410, 1973

29. Hart G: Sociological determinants of venereal disease, Br J Vener Dis 49: 542, 1973

30. Usilton LJ, Bruyere PI, Bruyere MC: The frequency of positive serologic tests for syphilis in relation to occupation and marital status among men of draft age, J Vener Dis Inform 26: 216, 1945

31. Watts GO, Wilson RA: A study of personality factors among venereal disease patients, Can Med Assoc J 53: 119, 1945

32. Campbell DJ: Venereal diseases in the armed forces overseas, Br J Vener Dis 22: 158, 1946

33. Olansky S, Simpson L, Schuman SH: Environmental factors in the Tuskegee study of untreated syphilis, Public Health Rep 69: 691, 1954

34. Wheldon GR: A poor man's Kinsey, J R Nav Med Serv 50: 109, 1964

35. Clark EG: Studies on syphilis in the Eastern Health District of Baltimore City, AM J Syph Gonor Vener Dis 29: 455, 1945

36. Ekstrom K: Patterns of sexual behavior in relation to venereal disease, Br J Vener Dis 46:93, 1970

37. Singh K, Mohamed E, Sukhija CL: Psychosocial background of servicemen contracting venereal diseases, J Indian Med Ass 46: 270, 1966

38. Clark T: The incidence, sociological aspects and suggestions as to the prevention of gonorrheal infections, South Med J 24: 691, 1931

39. Bundesen HN, Plotke F, Eisenberg H: Psychosomatic approach to venereal disease control, Am J Public Health 39: 1535, 1949

40. Weitz RD, Rachlin HL: The mental ability and educational attainment of five hundred venereally infected females, J Soc Hyg 31: 300, 1945

41. Ahrenfeldt RH: Psychiatry in the British army in the second world war, Routledge Kegan Paul, London, 1958

42. Belding DL, Hunter IL: The Wasserman test, Am J Syph 8: 117, 1924

43. Koch RA, Wilbur RL: Promiscuity as a factor in the spread of venereal disease, [Suppl. 20] J Vener Dis Inform 26: 144, 1945

44. Deschin CS: Teenagers and venereal disease: a sociological study of 600 teenagers in New York City social hygiene clinics, Am Soc Health Assoc, New York, 1961

45. Juhlin L: Factors influencing the spread of venereal disease, Acta Derm Venereal (Stockh) 48: 82, 1968

46. Keighley E: Immaturity and venereal disease in teenage girls Br J Vener Dis 39: 278, 1963

47. Willcox RR: A study of non specific urethritis in British soldiery, J Vener Dis Inform 30: 243, 1949

48. Donohue JF, Gleeson GA, Jenkins KH, Price EV: Venereal disease among teenagers—its relationship to juvenile delinquency, Public Health Rep 70: 453, 1955

49. Ingraham NR, Burke MJ: Juvenile delinquency and venereal disease among public school children in Philadelphia, J Vener Dis Inform 29: 362, 1948

50. Hart G: The relationship of personality to other sociological determinants of venereal disease, Br J Vener Dis 49: 548, 1973

51. Lion EG, Jambor HM, Corrigan HG, Bradway KP: An experiment in the psychiatric treatment of promiscuous girls, Venereal Disease Division, San Francisco Dept Public Health, 1945

52. Hart G Factors influencing venereal infection in wartime, Br J Vener Dis 50: 68, 1974

53. Larimore GW, Sternberg TH: Does health education prevent venereal disease?, Am J Public Health 35: 799, 1945

54. Editorial: The teenager and V.D., Am J Public Health 59: 898, 1969

55. Buck CW, Hobbs GE: The patient's attitude toward venereal disease education, J Vener Dis Inform 31: 204, 1950

56. Wann MD: A study of attitudes and informational levels with respect to gonorrhea, J Vener Dis Inform 24: 358, 1943

57. Hart G: Social and psychological aspects of venereal disease in Papua New Guinea, Br J Vener Dis 50: 453, 1974

58. Johns HM: The social aspects of the venereal diseases, Br J Vener Dis 21: 17, 1945

59. Beveridge MM: Source of infection with gonorrhoea in various ethnic groups, Br J Vener Dis 38: 154, 1962

60. Fiumara NJ: Venereal disease contacts of servicemen in Massachusetts, 1945–55, Public Health Rep 72: 455, 1957

61. Norris EW, Doyle AF, Iskrant AP: Venereal disease epidemiology Third Service Command: an analysis of 4,641 contact reports, Am J Public Health 33: 1065, 1943

62. Pemberton J, McCann JS, Mahony JDH, MacKenzie G, Dougan H, Hay I: Socio-medical characteristics of patients attending a V.D. clinic and the circumstances of infection, Br J Vener Dis 48: 391, 1972

63. Schofield M: The sexual behavior of young people, Longman's, London, 1965

64. Fiumara NJ: Effectiveness of condoms in preventing V.D., N Engl J Med 285: 972, 1971

65. McCormack WM, Lee Y, Zinner SH: Sexual experience and urethral colonization with genital mycoplasmas, Ann Intern Med 78: 696, 1973

66. Dudley S: The prevention of venereal disease in the Royal Navy, J R Nav Med Serv 53: 39, 1967

67. Hart G: Role of preventive methods in the control of venereal disease, Clin Obstet Gynecol 18: 243, 1975

68. Bennett FJ: The social determinants of gonorrhoea in an East African town, East Afr Med J 39: 332, 1962

69. Arya OP, Bennett FJ: Attitudes of college students in East Africa to sexual activity and venereal disease, Br J Vener Dis 44: 160, 1968

70. Dunham GC: Military preventive medicine, Telegraph Press, Pennsylvania, 1930

71. Cutler JC: Prophylaxis in the venereal diseases, Med Clin North Am 56: 1211, 1972

72. Walker AS: Clinical problems of war, Halstead Press, Sydney, 1952

73. Bettley FR: The medical conduct of a brothel, Br J Vener Dis 25: 56, 1949

74. Lees R: Venereal disease in the armed forces overseas, Br J Vener Dis 22: 149, 1946

75. Babione RW, Hedgecock LE, Ray JP: Navy experiences with oral use of penicillin as prophylaxis, US Armed Forces Med J 3: 973, 1952

76. Campbell VWH, Dougherty WJ, Curtis CE: Delayed administration of oral penicillin as prophylaxis for gonorrhea, Am J Syph 33: 437, 1949

77. Eagle H: Prevention of gonorrhea with penicillin tablets; preliminary report, Public Health Rep 63: 1411, 1948

Chapter Nine—Psychological Aspects of Venereal Disease

1. Watts GO, Wilson RA: A study of personality factors among venereal disease patients, Can Med Assoc J, 53: 119, 1945

2. Ratcliffe TA: Psychiatric and allied aspects of the problem of venereal disease in the army: with particular reference to S.E.A.C., J R Army Med Cps 89: 122, 1947

3. Wittkower ED, Cowan J: Some psychological aspects of sexual promiscuity, Psychosom Med, 6: 287, 1944

4. Eysenck HJ, Eysenck SBG: Manual of the Eysenck personality inventory, University of London Press, London, 1964

5. Eysenck HJ, Eysenck SBG: Scores on three personality variables as a function of age, sex and social class, Br J Soc Clin Psychol 8: 69, 1969

6. Eysenck HJ: Personality and sexual behavior, J Psychosom Res 16: 144, 1972

7. Giese H, Schmidt G: Studenten sexualitat, Rowholt, Hamburg, 1968

8. Wells BWP: Personality characteristics of V.D. patients, Br J Soc Clin Psychol 7: 286, 1969

9. Wells BWP: Personality study of V.D. patients using the psychoticism, extroversion, neuroticism inventory, Br J Vener Dis, 46: 498, 1970

10. Wells BWP, Schofield CBS: Personality characteristics of homosexual men suffering from sexually transmitted diseases, Br J Vener Dis 48: 75, 1972

11. Hart G: Psychological aspects of venereal disease in a war environment, Soc Sci Med 7: 455, 1973

12. Hart G: The relationship of personality to other sociological determinants of venereal disease, Br J Vener Dis 49: 548, 1973

13. Gibbens TCN: Prostitutes' and their clients' perception of venereal disease, in Ellis A, Abarbanel A: Encyclopedia of sexual behavior, 438 Corsano, London, 1962

14. Boneff AN: Psychopathology in V.D. practice, Indian J Dermatol 16: 51, 1971

15. Wessell MA, Pinck BD: Venereal disease anxiety, J Ment Hyg 31: 636, 1947

16. Hart G: The impact of prostitution on Australian troops at war, unpubl doctoral thesis, U Adelaide, South Australia, 1974

17. Wittkower ED: The psychological aspects of venereal disease, Br J Vener Dis 24: 59, 1948

18. Hart G: Psychosocial aspects of venereal disease in Papua New Guinea, Br J Vener Dis, 50: 453, 1974

19. Seth TR: Reaction of patients towards V.D. infection, Indian J Dermat Vener 36: 122, 1970

20. Henriques F: Modern sexuality, 243, Panther, London, 1969

21. Henriques F: The immoral tradition, 197, Panther, London, 1966

22. Lal S, Nicholas C: Epidemiological and clinical features in 165 cases of granuloma inguinale, Br J Vener Dis 46: 461, 1970

23. Maddocks I: Donovanosis in Papua, New Guinea Med J 10: 49, 1967

24. Pratt D: Personal communication, data from Indian Health Service, Window Rock, Arizona, 1975

25. Jacobs NF, Kraus SJ: Gonococcal and nongonococcal urethritis, Ann Intern Med 872: 7–12, 1975

26. Blount J: Personal communication, data from HSM 9.54, HEW, 1975

27. Holmes KK, Counts GW, Beatty HN: Disseminated gonococcal infection, Ann Intern Med 74: 979, 1971

28. Pahmer M: Psychiatric implications of venereal disease. An American survey, Br J Vener Dis 25: 124, 1949

29. Menninger K: A psychiatrist's world, Viking Press, New York, 1959

30. Mbanefo SE: Emotional problems of gonorrhea, J R Coll Gen Pract 15: 272, 1968

31. Datt I: Psychosocial aspects of venereal disease in teenagers, Indian J Dermatol 16: 27, 1971

32. Ellis A: Sexual manifestations of emotionally disturbed behavior, Am Acad Pol Soc Sci 376: 96, 1968

33. Rogerson HL: Venereophobia in the male, Br J Vener Dis 27: 158, 1951

34. Kite E de C, Grimble A: Psychiatric aspects of venereal disease, Br J Vener Dis 39: 1973, 1963

35. Faull DC: Venereophobia, Brit Med J 5234: 1247, 1961

36. Thyne GG: Venereophobia, Brit Med J 5220: 206, 1961

37. Dawid I: Venereophobia, Brit Med J 5224: 507, 1961

38. Pedder JR: Psychiatric referral of patients in a venereal disease clinic, Br J Vener Dis 46: 54, 1970

39. Hart G: The impact of prostitution on Australian troops at war, unpubl doctoral thesis, U Adelaide, South Australia, 1974

40. Giard R: Male gonococcal urethritis and its psychoemotional effects, Postgrad Med J, [January Suppl] 47, 1972

41. Macalpine I: Syphilophobia. A psychiatric study, Br J Vener Dis 33: 92, 1957

42. Atwater JB: Adapting the venereal disease clinic to today's problem, Am J Public Health, 64: 433-37, 1974

Chapter Ten—Special Groups

1. Ehrmann W: Social determinants of human sexual behavior, in Winokur G., Determinants of human sexual behavior, CC Thomas, Springfield, p. 142.

2. World Health Organization: International work in endemic treponematoses and venereal infections 1948-1963, 3. Gonococcal infections, WHO Chron 19: 7, 1965

3. Idsoe O, Kiraly K, Causse G: Venereal disease and treponematoses—the epidemiologic situation and WHO's control program, WHO Chron 27: 410, 1973

4. Editorial: Immigrants and venereal disease, Br Med J 3: 129, 1969

5. Willcox RR: Immigration and venereal disease in England and Wales, Br J Vener Dis 46: 412, 1970

6. Verhagen AR, Gemert W: Social and epidemiological determi-

nants of gonorrhea in an East African country, Br J Vener Dis 48: 277, 1972

7. Hart G: Psychosocial aspects of venereal disease in Papua New Guinea, Br J Vener Dis 50: 453, 1974

8. Brown WJ, Donohue JF, Axnick NW, Blount JH, Ewen NH, Jones OG: Syphilis and the other venereal diseases, Harvard University Press, Massachusetts, 1970

9. Hart G: Sociological determinants of venereal disease, Br J Vener Dis 49: 542, 1973

10. Hinrichsen J: Venereal disease in the major armies and navies of the world, J Syph Gonor Vener Dis 28: 736, 1944

11. Greenberg JH: Venereal disease in the armed forces, Med Clin North Am 56: 1087, 1972

12. Havard V: Manual of military medicine, William Wood Co, New York, 1909

13. Witkower Ed, Cowan J: Some psychological aspects of sexual promiscuity, Psychosom Med 6: 287, 1944

14. Ahrenfeldt RH: Psychiatry in the British army in the second world war, Routledge Kegan Paul, London, 1958

15. Ratcliffe TA: Psychiatric and allied aspects of the problem of venereal disease in the army: with particular reference to S.E.A.C., J R Army Med Cps 89: 122, 1947

16. Singh K, Mohamed E, Sukhija CL: Psychosocial background of servicemen contracting venereal diseases, J Indian Med Assoc 46: 270, 1966

17. Butler AG: Official history of the Australian army medical services 1914-18, Vol. III, Problems and services, Australian War Memorial, Canberra, 1943

18. Dunham GC: Military preventive medicine, Telegraph Press, Pennsylvania, 1930

19. Stouffer SA, Suchman EA, De Vinney LC, Star SA, Williams RM: The American soldier, Wiley, New York, 1965

20. Barber N: The war of the running dogs, 120, Collins, London, 1971

21. Cooperman RS: VD in Vietnam, N Engl J Med 283: 546, 1970

22. Ross AOF: The different aspects of maritime venereal disease control, Rotterdam Port Demonstration Center, 1953-1954 WHO Publ, 1956

23. Hermans EH: Interrelationship of syphilis incidence and maritime activity, World forum on syphilis and other treponematoses, Public Health Rep 997, 1962

Chapter Eleven—Failure to Control Venereal Disease

1. Idsoe O, Kiraly K, Causse G: Venereal disease and treponematoses—the epidemiologic situation and WHO's control program. WHO Chron 27: 410, 1973

2. Gilbert DN, Greenberg JH: Vietnam: preventive medicine orientation, Milit Med 132: 769, 1967

3. Willcox RR: Prostitution and venereal disease, Antiseptic 60: 1, 1963

4. Lomholt G, Berg O: Gonorrhoea situation in South Greenland in the summer of 1964, Br J Vener Dis 42: 1, 1966

5. Guthe T, Willcox RR: The international incidence of venereal disease, Int Health Conf, Edinburgh, 1970

6. Donohue JF: Problems posed by population mobility in control of syphilis, Proc World Forum on Syphilis and Other Treponematoses, Public Health Rep 997, 1964

Chapter Twelve—Controlling Venereal Infection

1. Australian Medical Association: Report of the Federal Coordinating Committee on the problem of venereal disease in Australia, Med J Aust, [Suppl] 3: 17, 1967

2. Jenkins CD: The epidemiology of public response, Proc 6th Annual Immun Conf Public Health Rep 115–118, 1969

3. Greenberg, JH: Venereal disease in the armed forces, Med Clin N Amer 56: 1087, 1972

4. Harrison WO, et al: Prevention of gonorrhea. Evaluation of prophylactic antibiotics. Presented at 13th Intersci Conf Antimicrobial Agents and Chemotherapy, Washington, 19–21, 1973

5. Hackett CJ, Guthe T: Some important aspects of yaws eradication, Bull WHO 15: 869–96, 1956

6. Hinman EH: The world eradication of infectious diseases, 52, CC Thomas, Springfield, 1966

7. U.S. Department Health, Education and Welfare, Syphilis epidemiology, report 10, Publication No. (HSM), 72–8097, 1970

8. Frye WW: The importance of contact investigation in the control of syphilis, Med Clin North Am 48: 637, 1964

9. Wigfield AS: 27 years of uninterrupted contact tracing. The Tyneside scheme, Br J Vener Dis 48: 37, 1972

10. Hare MJ, Lamb AM, King DM: Contact tracing in gonorrhea, Br J Vener Dis 46: 485, 1970

11. Macfarlane WV: Further observation on the medicosocial aspects of venereal disease, Public Health. 62: 4, 1948
12. Lamb AM: New methods of contact tracing in infectious venereal diseases, Br J Vener Dis 42: 276, 1966
13. Blount BA: A new approach to gonorrhea epedemiology, Am J Public Health 62: 710, 1972

Index

Abortion. *See* Pregnancy, termination
Abscess, 110, 112
Abstinence, 33, 155, 161
Adolescents. *See* Teenagers
Adoption, 41
Age, 6, 27–29, 31, 45, 79, 83, 84, 97,
    129, 142–45, 154, 173, 186, 197
Aggression, 16, 79, 125, 148,
    158, 188
Alcohol, 65, 68, 71, 126, 134–36, 138,
    143–45, 151, 158, 162
Allergy, to penicillin, 91, 192
Alopecia, 101
Amoxicillin, 91, 190
Ampicillin, 91, 116, 120, 190
Anal intercourse, 31–35, 79
Animals, 114, 188. *See also*
    Behavior, animal
Antibiotics, 147, 149, 151, 168, 169,
    177, 181, 190–92, 194. *See also*
    Amoxicillin; Ampicillin;
    Chloramphenicol; Gentamycin
    Kanamycin; Penicillin;
    Tetracyclines
Apathy, 146, 147, 152, 195, 196,
    200, 203

Armed forces. *See* Military
Arthritis, 88, 147
Asymptomatic states, 17, 35, 36, 79,
    86, 87, 89, 92, 95, 98, 99, 107,
    113, 116, 149, 159, 171, 182–85,
    187, 198, 204
Attitudes, 5–18, 20, 21, 29, 37, 44–46,
    49–53, 62, 128, 132–34, 137, 138,
    146–52, 155, 158, 160, 170, 171,
    195–97
Australia, 27, 125, 127, 128, 133–40,
    144, 158, 159, 175, 176
Autoeroticism. *See* Masturbation

Balanitis, 83, 120, 121
Bartholin's gland, 86
Behavior, 52, 155, 158, 164, 173, 195,
    204. *See also under names of*
    specific behaviors
    animal, 19, 30, 54, 75, 76
    health-seeking, 4, 18, 195, 196
    homosexual, 73–80, 156, 183
    intimate, 49, 77
    sexual, 12–37, 53, 69, 123, 142, 154,
    155, 161
Benzathine penicillin. *See* Penicillin

Benzene hexachloride, 114, 115
Benzyl benzoate, 114, 115
Biologic false-positive tests. *See*
    False-positive tests
Birth control. *See* Pregnancy,
    prophylaxis
Bisexual, 73, 74
Blood tests. *See* Serologic tests
Brothel, 53–72, 139, 140, 161, 162.
    See also Prostitution; War

Caesarean section, 45, 96, 107
Candidiasis, 1, 2, 82, 83, 116, 82, 83,
    119–21, 181, 182
  diagnosis, 121
  etiologic factors, 119–21
  treatment, 121
Case record, 164, 177–81
Casefinding, 133, 163, 169, 171, 181,
    183, 193–200
Cephalothin, 110
Chancre, 99, 101
Chancroid, 1, 2, 4, 8, 82, 109–11
  clinicopathological features, 109, 110
  diagnosis, 110
  history, 109
  treatment, 110, 111
Children, 33, 40, 45, 106, 118, 148,
    173, 191
Chlamydia, 2, 92, 111
Chloramphenicol, 109
Circumcision, 29, 34
Clinics, 1, 4–9, 17, 27, 44, 82, 152,
    155, 164, 168–70, 177–81, 196,
    202. *See also* Health services
Cluster interview, 197–200
Coitus, 1, 20, 26–36, 38–47, 111, 128,
    134, 153, 155, 161
  age of first, 27, 142, 144, 158
  premarital, 17, 20
Coitus interruptus. *See* Withdrawal
College students, 27–32, 86, 137, 138,
    147
Complacency, 160, 168, 169
Complement fixation tests. *See*
    Serologic tests
Complications
  of IUD, 40
  of therapy, 91, 140, 181, 193, 194

of VD, 2, 4, 7, 147, 172, 194
Condom, 38, 39, 97, 136–40, 196
Condyloma acuminatum, 2, 4, 34, 35,
    82, 83, 116–18, 150, 183
  clinical features, 117
  diagnosis, 117
  history, 116, 117
  pathology, 117
  treatment, 117, 118
Condylomata lata, 101
Congenital syphilis. *See* Syphilis
Conjunctivitis, 87, 88, 92
Contact tracing. *See* Casefinding
Contacts. *See* Partners, sexual
Contraception. *See* Pregnancy,
    prophylaxis
Control of venereal disease, 1, 4–9,
    59–61, 72, 79, 80, 136, 140, 153,
    161, 162, 164, 167–204
Corynebacterium vaginale infection,
    2, 4, 115, 116
  clinical features, 116
  diagnosis, 116
  treatment, 116
Covert homosexuals, 74
Crime, 133, 142–45, 148, 157, 158
    See also Laws
Cunnilingus, 95, 111, 142. *See also*
    Orogenital sex
Cytomegalovirus infection, 2, 4, 84,
    106, 107, 183, 191

Darkfield microscopy, 97, 101, 102
Depression, 150
Developing countries, 5, 6, 56, 70, 104,
    118, 127, 146, 156, 167, 191, 192
Diagnosis, 5, 151, 176. *See also*
    Candidiasis; Chancroid;
    Condyloma acuminatum;
    Cytomgalovirus infection;
    Donovanosis; Gonorrhea;
    Lymphogranuloma venereum;
    Molluscum contagiosum;
    Nongonococcal urethritis;
    Pediculosis pubis; Scabies;
    Syphilis; Trichomoniasis
Discharge. *See* Gonococcal infection;
    Nongonococcal urethritis;
    Vaginitis

Distribution, 157, 183
Doctors, 4–18, 20, 37, 41–47, 59–61,
    78, 82, 149–52, 155, 157, 168–70,
    175, 176, 197, 200
Donovanosis, 1, 2, 4, 8, 33, 34, 80, 82,
    107–9, 146, 156, 157, 182
  clinicopathological features,
    107, 108
  diagnosis, 108, 109
  history, 107
  treatment, 109
Drugs, 21, 68, 104, 143, 158. *See also*
    Treatment; *under names of*
    specific drugs
Dyspareunia, 10, 53, 120

Education, 11–18, 27, 28, 63, 128, 130,
    131, 143–45, 152, 157, 168, 175,
    186, 192, 200
Emotion, 16, 53, 54, 66, 76, 149
Environment, 123–26, 129, 132, 135,
    142, 145, 158, 182, 183, 188, 189
Epidemiologic treatment. *See*
    Treatment, epidemiologic
Epidemiology, 83, 133, 168, 169,
    176, 181–204
Eroticism, 30, 64, 69, 73, 74
Erythromycin, 106
Extragenital infection. *See*
    Conjunctivitis; Pharyngitis;
    Perihepatitis; Proctitis
Extramarital sex, 17, 30. 142
Extroversion, 27, 52, 142–52

Fallopian tube, 86
False-positive tests, 104, 186, 187
Family, 27, 123, 132, 158, 170
Fear, 12, 14, 140. 142, 148, 150, 152,
    154, 159, 160, 168
Fellatio, 35, 57, 65, 73, 79, 95, 131,
    142, 144, 161. *See also* Orogenital
    sex
Female. *See* Women
Flagyl. *See* Metronidazole
Fluorescent treponemal antibody-
    absorption test (FTA-ABS). *See*
    Serologic tests
Frei test, 112

Gentamycin, 109

Giemsa stain, 96–98, 107, 108, 121
Gonococcal infection, 2, 82–93, 106,
    147
  anorectal infection, 87, 183
  conjunctivitis, 87, 88, 92
  diagnosis, 89, 90
  disseminated infection, 88, 92
  endocervicitis, 86
  history, 84, 85
  pathology, 85
  pelvic inflammatory disease, 86, 87
  perihepatitis, 87
  pharyngitis, 87, 182
  treatment, 91, 92
  urethritis, 85, 86
Gonorrhea, ix, 1, 4–10, 17, 18, 33–36,
    105, 127–40, 153–60, 167–73,
    181–87, 190, 193, 194, 204. *See*
    also Gonococcal infection
Gram stain, 89–93, 110, 116, 121, 149,
    194, 195
Granuloma inguinale. *See*
    Donovanosis
Guilt, 12, 14, 20, 44, 126, 133, 142,
    144, 147, 148, 170

Health services, 4–10, 128, 176–81,
    195–97. *See also* Clinics
Hemophilus ducreyi, 2, 34, 109, 110.
    See also Chancroid
Hemophilus vaginalis. See
    Corynebacterium vaginale
    infection
Hepatitis, 104, 181, 182
Herpes genitalis. *See* Herpes
    simplex infection
Herpes simplex infection, 2, 4, 33–36,
    82–84, 94–97, 107, 183, 191
  clinicopathological features, 94, 95
  diagnosis, 95, 96
  epidemiologic features, 95
  history, 94
  HSV–1, 94, 95
  HSV–2, 2, 94–96
  management, 96, 97
Heterosexual, 50, 73, 74, 76, 142, 157.
    183–85
High risk groups, 4, 84, 127–40,
    153–65, 172, 183, 195, 196

History, 6–8. *See also* Chancroid;
    Condyloma acuminatum;
    Corynebacterium vaginale
    infection; Cytomegalovirus
    infection; Donovanosis;
    Gonococcal infection;
    Lymphogranuloma venereum;
    Molluscum contagiosum;
    Nongonococcal urethritis;
    Pediculosis pubis; Scabies;
    Syphilis; Trichomoniasis
    medical, 14, 150, 151
Homosexual, 13, 16, 18, 30–32, 35, 50,
    65, 73–80, 84, 142, 183–85,
    196, 197
Homosexuality, 4, 73–80
Host factors, 119, 121

Illegitimate children, 41–46
Immigrants, 55, 123, 156, 157
Immunization, 172, 173, 190–92, 196
Immunofluorescence, 90, 101
Incidence, 19, 26–36, 187
    of homosexuality, 75
    of venereal diseases, 2, 4–7, 82, 153,
    157, 200
Income, 131
Infectivity, 83, 117, 199
Intelligence, 52–54, 63, 131
Intercourse. *See* Coitus
Intrauterine device (IUD), 38–40
Introversion, 142–52

Juvenile delinquency, 143

Kanamycin, 93, 110
Kissing, 95, 155

Laws, 43, 50, 61, 62, 69, 71, 72,
    77, 170, 192
Lice. *See* Pediculosis pubis
Lymphogranuloma venereum, 1, 2, 4,
    82, 111–13
    clinical features, 111, 112
    diagnosis, 112, 113
history, 111
    treatment, 113

Male. *See* Men

Marital status, 45, 129, 130
Marriage, 7, 12, 13, 17, 21, 28–30,
    41–47, 50, 51, 55, 65, 69, 71, 126,
    129, 158
Masturbation, 28–34, 50, 51, 57, 79,
    131, 134, 142, 144, 146, 148, 158
Medical services. *See* Clinics; Health
    services
Men, 20, 21, 26–36, 40, 44–46, 53,
    81–84, 147, 156, 181, 182, 198
Meningitis, 88
Menstruation, 37–47, 86, 97
Metronidazole, 93, 98
Migrants. *See* Immigrants
Military, 5–9, 27, 29, 31, 60, 61, 65,
    79, 123–42, 146, 157–63, 172–75,
    190, 191
Miscarriage. *See* Pregnancy,
    termination
Mobility, 163, 171, 186, 203
Molluscum contagiosum, 2, 4, 82,
    83, 118, 119, 182, 183
    clinical features, 118, 119
    diagnosis, 119
    epidemiology, 118
    history, 118
    management, 119
    pathology, 118
Monilia. *See* Candidiasis
Morality, 7–9, 50, 58, 59, 69, 71, 147,
    155, 159, 161
Morbidity, 4, 6, 181, 193
Mortality, 7, 41–45
Mycoplasma, 92, 137, 138

Neisseria gonorrhoeae, 85, 89. *See also*
    Gonococcal infection
Neonates, 94, 106, 120
Neurosyphilis, 7, 101
Neuroticism, 27, 76, 78, 81, 142–52,
    199
Nongonococcal urethritis, 4, 82–84,
    92–94, 146, 149, 195, 204
    diagnosis, 93
    management, 93, 94
Nonspecific urethritis. *See*
    Nongonococcal urethritis
Norms, 19, 20, 75–78, 123
Nystatin, 89, 121

Occupation, 131, 153–65
Ophthalmia neonatorum, 87, 88, 92,
    139. *See also* Conjunctivitis
Orgasm, 21, 30, 52, 57
Orogenital sex, 30–32, 35, 148. *See also*
    Cunnilingus; Fellatio
Oxidase reaction, 89

Papanicalaou smear, 39, 96, 107
Paraphimosis, 34
Parental influence, 43, 45, 46, 75, 76,
    132, 154–56
Partners, sexual, 17, 34, 40, 49, 52,
    77–79, 83, 84, 94, 97, 114, 118,
    129, 130, 148, 150, 156–58,
    195, 197–200
Pediculosis pubis, 2, 4, 82, 83, 113,
    114, 181, 182
  clinical features, 113
  diagnosis, 114
  pathology, 113
  treatment, 114
Pelvic inflammatory disease. *See*
    Gonococcal infection
Penicillin, 93, 168, 191, 192
  benzathine, 106
  crystalline, 91
  procaine, 91, 106
Penile ulcers, 82, 83. *See also*
    Chancroid; Donovanosis;
    Herpes simplex; Syphilis
Penis, 29, 38, 93, 148–51
Perihepatitis, 87
Permissive society, 50
Personality, 45, 50–53, 128, 133, 135,
    141–52, 155, 160
Pharyngitis, 33, 35, 84, 91, 183–85
Physicians. *See* Doctors
Pill, contraceptive, 38–40, 53, 120, 168
Podophyllin, 117
Pregnancy, 21, 29, 30, 66, 84, 98,
    104, 106, 117–19, 194
  prophylaxis, 5, 10, 20, 30, 37–41.
    See also Intrauterine device; Pill,
    contraceptive; Rhythm method;
    Sterilization
  termination, 41–47
    complications, 44
    techniques, 43, 44

  unwanted, 4, 17, 18, 37–47, 50
    assessment, 44–46
    complications, 43
    management, 41–46
Prejudice, 7–9, 19, 66–69, 173, 203
Prevalence, 4, 171, 185–87, 207
Prevention. *See* Prophylaxis
Prisons, 8, 78, 79
Probenecid, 91
Proctitis, 84, 183–85
Promiscuity, 4, 18, 27, 49–72, 79,
    123–27, 129–40, 154–64, 170, 186
  definition, 49
  habitual, 49–53, 142, 146
  transient, 49–53
Prophylaxis, 4, 59, 131, 135–40, 151,
    164, 173, 190, 191. *See also*
    Condom; Pill, contraceptive;
    Pregnancy, prophylaxis
Prostitutes, 27, 28, 32, 73, 95, 127–40,
    147, 150, 156, 161, 162, 170, 171,
    188, 197. *See also* Prostitution
Prostitution, 4, 49–72, 144, 145, 157
  definition, 53–55
  regulation, 59–62
  types 55–58
  VD and, 59–62, 69–72, 124–26
Psychological aspects, 7–10, 12, 20, 21,
    30, 40–47, 50–53, 68, 77, 121,
    130, 141–52, 169
Psychotic, 150, 151
Punishment, 7–9, 158–63

Quarantine, 188–90

Race, 33, 43, 86, 97, 128, 130, 147,
    156, 157, 187, 197
Rapid plasma reagin (RPR) test.
    See Serologic tests
Rashes, 101, 104, 115
Recidivism, 4, 159, 173, 177, 186
Rectal coitus. *See* Anal intercourse
Rectal infection. *See* Proctitis
Reiter protein complement fixation
    test. *See* Serologic tests
Reiter's disease, 146
Reliability, of patient, 39, 53, 91, 133
Religion, 27, 46, 58, 134, 154, 156,
    170, 175

Reporting, 5, 6, 167, 200
Research, 13, 42
Reservoir of infection, 170, 171, 199
Rhythm method, 38
Risk of infection, 129, 183, 194

Salpingitis. *See* Pelvic inflammatory
    disease
Scabies, 2, 4, 82, 83, 114, 115, 181, 182
    clinical features, 115
    diagnosis, 115
    pathology, 114, 115
    treatment, 115
Screening, 103–5, 128, 133, 147, 161,
    167, 183–87, 192–95, 199, 202–4
Seamen, 65, 70, 79, 123, 163, 164, 172
Sensitivity, 90, 91, 103–5, 183–87, 193
Serologic tests, 102–5, 171, 186, 187,
    192, 204
    complement fixation
        for LGV, 112
        for syphilis, 102
    fluorescent treponemal antibody-
        absorption (FTA-ABS) test, 102–5
    FTA-ABS-IgM, 102–3
    Kahn, 102
    Kolmer, 102
    rapid plasma reagin (RPR), 102
    Reiter protein complement fixation
        test (RPCFT), 102
    Treponema pallidum
        hemagglutination ,TPHA), 102
    Treponema pallidum
        immobilization (TPI), 99–105
    venereal disease research
        laboratory (VDRL), 100–5
    Wassermann, 99, 102
Sex, 11–18. *See also* Men; Women
Sexual intercourse. *See* Coitus
Shame, 12, 14, 126, 133, 142, 148, 170
Silver nitrate, 138, 139
Smallpox, 191, 192
Socioeconomic status, 21, 45, 50, 95,
    99, 128, 131, 132, 196, 197
Soft sore. *See* Chancroid
Specificity, 90, 102–5, 183–87, 193
Spectinomycin, 91
Standards, 56, 69, 71, 123
Statistics, 5–7, 126, 127, 153, 154, 162,

167, 177. *See also* Incidence;
    Prevalence
Sterility, 17
Sterilization, 38–41, 45
Streptomycin, 109, 110
Stres, 27, 123–26, 150, 156, 157, 160,
    163
Sulfisoxazole, 110, 113
Surveillance, 151, 177, 194, 196
Symptoms. *See* Asymptomatic states;
    under names of specific diseases
Syphilis, 1, 2, 4–9, 13, 17, 33–36, 80,
    82–84, 98–107, 110, 128–40, 146,
    147, 154, 156, 157, 167, 168,
    171–73, 183, 191, 195, 197–200,
    204
    clinical features, 99–101
    congenital, 99
    diagnosis, 101–5
    history, 99
    late, 100–6
    latent, 100–6
    primary, 99–105
    secondary, 100–5
    serology (*see* False-positive tests;
        Serologic tests)
    treatment, 105, 106

Teenagers, 6, 40, 65, 75, 136, 153–56,
    196
Tetracyclines, 91–93, 106, 109, 110,
    113, 120, 190
Thayer-Martin medium, 89, 90, 93
Titer, 102–5, 107, 112
Transmission (sexual), 1, 4, 33, 94,
    97, 99, 106, 113, 114, 116, 181
Treatment, 5–9, 11, 14, 78, 177, 181.
    *See also under names of specific
    diseases*
    abortive, 177
    epidemiologic, 177, 194–95, 202–4
    mass, 191, 192, 194, 195
    prophylactic, 177
Treponema pallidum, 33, 98–104
Treponema pallidum hemagglutination
    test. *See* Serologic tests
Treponema pallidum immobilization
    test. *See* Serologic tests
Trichomoniasis, 1, 2, 4, 82–84, 97,

98, 116, 119
    clinicopathologic aspects, 97
    diagnosis, 97, 98
    epidemiology, 97
    history, 97
    management, 98
Tubal ligation. *See* Sterilization
Tzanck smear, 96

Ulcers, 101, 107, 109, 195. *See also*
    Penile ulcers
Underdeveloped countries. *See*
    Developing countries
Urban populations, 167
Urethritis, 82, 169, 204. *See also*
    Gonorrhea; Nongonococcal
    urethritis

Vaccine. *See* Immunization
Vaginitis, 97, 120, 121
Venereal disease research laboratory
    (VDRL). *See* Serologic tests

Venereoneurosis, 140, 148–52
Vietnam, 27, 31, 127–40, 144, 158,
    159, 161

War, 5–8, 27, 56, 66, 114, 123–40,
    158–63, 188. *See also* Military;
    Vietnam
Warts (genital). *See* Condyloma
    acuminatum
Withdrawal, 38
Women, 6, 20, 21, 27–47, 67, 82–84,
    94–98, 147, 154, 156, 160, 170,
    171, 182, 183, 198
World Health Organization (WHO),
    5, 191
Wright's stain, 108, 121

Xylocaine, 96

Yaws, 99, 191, 192
Yield, 35, 59, 128, 172, 193–95, 202–3

Zinc oxide, 96